A LABORATORY GUIDE TO
THE ANATOMY OF THE RABBIT

A Laboratory Guide to the
ANATOMY OF THE RABBIT

BY

E. HORNE CRAIGIE

Professor of Comparative Anatomy and Neurology
University of Toronto

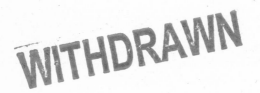

SECOND EDITION

UNIVERSITY OF TORONTO PRESS
TORONTO

Printed in Canada by
University of Toronto Press
Toronto and Buffalo

PREFACE

AFTER many years of teaching mammalian anatomy the author is more than ever convinced of the advantages of the rabbit as a type for student dissection.

The present work does not in any way aim to replace *Bensley's Practical Anatomy of the Rabbit,* which has long since proved its value beyond question. The attempt has been to meet a need for a shorter and less detailed laboratory guide adapted to courses for which *Bensley's Anatomy* has been found too extensive. Classes for which the present book is designed have assignments of time for this subject varying from about twenty-four hours to about sixty hours. Some of them have two-hour periods and some have three-hour periods. Some, moreover, have need for special emphasis on certain parts which are of less immediate interest to others.

Hence it was felt undesirable from every point of view to prepare a text fitted to one particular course. Rather the aim has been to present a reasonably brief account in such a way that an instructor can assign from it the chapters most suited for a particular class and can easily omit parts which he feels less important or which his time-schedule does not allow him to include. At the same time the occasional student with sufficient curiosity can extend his study beyond class assignments.

For a more complete account the curious student would naturally have to turn to *Bensley's Practical Anatomy* and the present author has inevitably leaned heavily upon that work, his indebtedness to which he gladly acknowledges.

In the hope of making it easier for beginning students to integrate the parts studied in their minds and to understand the body as a living, working mechanism, an attempt has been made to arrange the presentation so as to bring together wherever practicable the different parts of each organ system, these being inevitably somewhat scattered in the strict regional method of dissection. The inter-relations of systems, which are more high-lighted by the latter method, are nevertheless still kept in view. Although the current term "functional anatomy" is not used, it is hoped that the essence of this very fundamental concept has been kept before the dissector. Some modified approaches in dissection have been introduced with this aim.

Of the twenty-eight illustrations, fifteen are new and the remainder have been borrowed from *Bensley's Practical Anatomy*. Four of the latter were the work of the late Dr. Bensley, the rest were prepared by the present author.

For permission to use illustrations as well as descriptive material from *Bensley's Practical Anatomy* the author is grateful to the University of Toronto Press, which owns the copyright for that work. He is also grateful for the co-operation of the Press in preparation of this new text-book.

E. Horne Craigie

Toronto, December, 1950

CONTENTS

A LABORATORY GUIDE TO
THE ANATOMY OF THE RABBIT

CHAPTER I

MICROSCOPIC ANATOMY

STUDY of the structure of the bodies of animals is commonly divided into microscopic anatomy and gross anatomy. This classification, however, is based merely upon the sizes of the parts to be examined and the consequent need of somewhat different technical methods of study. The two are essentially one in outlook and they are equally essential for an understanding of the structure, a knowledge of which is a prerequisite for any intelligent study of functions, of behaviour, of development, of diseases, and so on.

The present work is to be concerned with gross anatomy, but in view of the considerations just suggested an introductory glance at some fundamentals of microscopic structure appears to be desirable.

The basic unit of living matter, both structurally and functionally, is a cell. Though this can be further analyzed, none of its component parts can be regarded in the same ways as a complete living unit. Each cell consists of a mass of living, jelly-like, protein material, protoplasm, which comprises an inner, differentiated nucleus and a surrounding layer of cytoplasm. The surface of the cytoplasm forms a cell-membrane and within it various other structural elements often appear (Fig. 1).

All animals except the simplest (protozoa) have many cells associated to form their bodies and usually there are marked differences among the cells in a single animal body as well as in the intercellular materials which hold them together. Cells of more or less similar character are assembled into tissues, in which they are held together by intercellular materials that vary greatly in amount and in nature but are characteristic for each type of tissue.

Tissues are associated in various ways to form organs. The definition of the word organ lacks precision but in general it is a part of the body devoted to some special function, such as digestion or respiration. The study of organs and of their larger assemblages, known as organ-systems, is the role of gross anatomy, while tissues and cells belong to microscopic anatomy, or histology.

In gross anatomy, however, it is necessary for the student to recognize the main types of tissues and their more important subdivisions. These main types are epithelial, connective, muscular, and nervous tissues, besides blood and lymph, which are sometimes classed as liquid tissues.

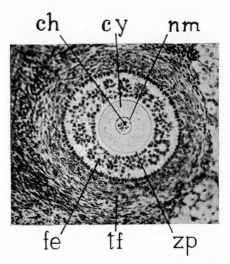

Fig. 1. Photomicrograph of a section of a developing ovum in the ovary of a rabbit. X150. From *Bensley's Practical Anatomy of the Rabbit*. ch, chromatin; cy, cytoplasm; fe, follicular epithelium; nm, nucleur membrane; tf, theca folliculi; zp, zona pellucida.

EPITHELIAL TISSUE

Epithelial tissue is the characteristic covering of free surfaces. It may be only one cell in thickness (simple epithelium) or may have many layers (stratified epithelium). Also it may produce a variety of secondary structures such as hairs, claws, etc. The amount of intercellular material present is relatively small.

Examples of simple epithelium are surface layers of the mesenteries and the lining of most parts of the alimentary canal. Stratified epithelium forms the outer part of the skin, the epidermis.

Specialized epithelium constitutes most (though not all) glands, the essential structure of which is either an assemblage of epithelial tubules or an assemblage of flask-shaped structures (acini) which are also epithelial. Such glands may either retain their connection with a free surface by a duct through which the secretion passes (exocrine glands) or lose this connection so that the secretion must be conveyed by the blood or lymph (endocrine glands). The various digestive glands are examples of the former, the thyreoid gland is an example of the latter. An example of an endocrine gland which is not epithelial is the suprarenal body.

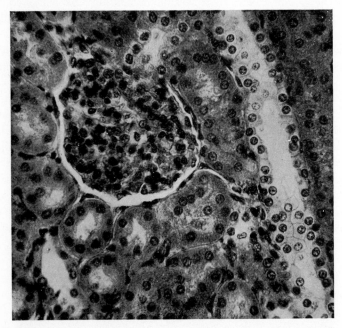

Fig. 2. Photomicrograph of a small part of a section of the kidney of a rabbit. X360. From *Bensley's Practical Anatomy of the Rabbit*. A collecting tubule running through the right third of the field shows the appearance of simple epithelium both in section and in surface view. A glomerulus appears in its Bowman's capsule, the latter lined by flattened epithelium, and the rest of the field contains mainly sections of convoluted tubules, which also illustrate simple cuboidal or low columnar epithelium.

Certain epithelia differ from the rest in that they are formed not over originally free surfaces but as linings of internal cavities developed within primarily continuous masses of embryonic tissue. According to location they are distinguished as mesothelium and endothelium. The lining of the peritoneal cavity, including the surfaces of the mesenteries mentioned above, is mesothelium, the lining of the blood-vessels is endothelium.

CONNECTIVE TISSUE

The general function of connective tissue is just what, in a broad sense, that term implies. Such tissue is characterized by the presence of a relatively large amount of intercellular material, the diversified nature of which distinguishes different varieties of connective tissue and confers upon them the properties which particularly fit them for their special rôles. These various types may be classified into ordinary or soft connective tissues and skeletal tissues (cartilage and bone).

The ordinary connective tissues have the cells scattered through an intercellular matrix (produced by the cells themselves) containing usually three kinds of fibres—white, yellow, and reticular—with a watery or viscid liquid between them. This is frequently known as fibrous connective tissue, its commonest variety being called areolar, exemplified by the loose white subcutaneous tissue which attaches the skin and by the fascia between muscles. The fibres of the matrix are interlaced in a felt-like manner. When these fibres are more numerous and concentrated, they may form a strong, tough sheet, as in the deeper layer of the skin, the corium. Still more compact and with the white fibres mostly parallel are the ligaments which hold bones together and the tendons which attach muscles to bones.

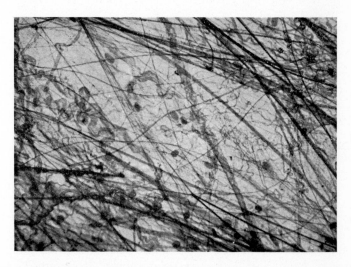

Fig. 3. Photomicrograph of part of a stained preparation of areolar connective tissue (subcutaneous tissue of a rabbit). X150. From *Bensley's Practical Anatomy of the Rabbit.*

Fat or adipose tissue differs from those just mentioned in that the matrix is quantitatively less than the cells and the latter are distended by large droplets of fat within their cytoplasm. The tissue derives from this substance an opaque white, yellow, or even brownish colour and a peculiar consistency.

The skeletal tissues have fewer fibres in the matrix but this matrix is largely solid instead of liquid, so that such tissues are suitable materials for the supporting framework of the body as well as for protective shields.

Cartilage is the more flexible type of skeletal tissue. Hyaline cartilage has an apparently homogeneous matrix with a certain amount of elasticity and a pale, translucent, blue-grey colour. It occurs in such places as the nose or the larynx and as a thin layer over the articular surfaces of bones in the joints. Fibrocartilage differs in that many white fibres are imbedded in the hyaline matrix, giving increased toughness. It occurs, for example, in the pelvic symphysis and at the margins of the capsules in joints. The epiglottic cartilage and that of the external ear, which are very flexible, contain many yellow fibres and exemplify elastic cartilage.

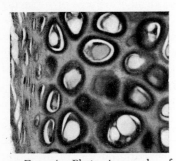

FIG. 4. Photomicrograph of part of a stained section of cartilage from the ear of a rabbit. X230. From *Bensley's Practical Anatomy of the Rabbit.*

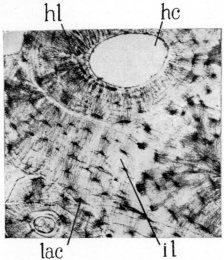

FIG. 5. Photomicrograph of part of a ground transverse section of the bone of a human radius. X120. From *Bensley's Practical Anatomy of the Rabbit.* hc, Haversian canal; hl, Haversian lamella; il, interstitial lamella; lac, lacuna.

Bone is a denser, harder, tissue with relatively little elasticity, its matrix being strengthened by the presence throughout of much inorganic material (mainly salts of calcium). Within the matrix, the cells lie within minute cavities, the lacunae, which are connected with each other by fine canaliculi and are arranged in definite patterns differing according to the manner of origin of the particular bone.

Developmentally, bone may replace cartilage, which is slowly eaten away while bone is formed in its stead—cartilage or replacing bone—or it may be produced directly in the soft connective tissue—membrane or derm bone. The adult tissue is the same in either case.

Most bones of the skeleton contain cavities filled with soft, highly vascular, connective tissue, the bone-marrow, which is the most important of several regions where red blood cells develop.

MUSCULAR TISSUE

Muscular tissue is the principal agent of movement in the body. It composes the active portions of the organs known as muscles and occurs in the constitution of many other organs where movement is required, as in the walls of the digestive tube and other visceral organs. The colour is usually reddish in the fresh condition though it may be quite pale. Red muscle acts more slowly and is less subject to fatigue than "white" muscle.

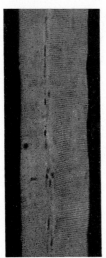

FIG. 6. Photomicrograph of parts of two striated-muscle fibres from a teased preparation of skeletal muscle of a rabbit. From *Bensley's Practical Anatomy of the Rabbit.*

Muscular tissue is characterized by the elongation of the individual cells into long, parallel fibres held together by a minimum of intercellular substance, these fibres having the primary protoplasmic function of contractility accentuated and restricted to the direction of their length. They are grouped in parallel bundles surrounded by small quantities of connective tissue and attached by tendon or directly to the points upon which they are to pull, these bundles often giving a muscle a very finely lined appearance.

The term striated muscle, however, refers not to the appearance just mentioned but to fine lines running across each fibre and visible only under the microscope. Such fibres constitute all the skeletal muscles and are usually under the control of the will, so are often called voluntary.

Smooth muscle, in contrast, has fibres which show no such markings and are usually shaped like much-elongated spindles, though shorter than striated fibres. They are involuntary and occur mainly in the walls of visceral organs and blood-vessels.

Cardiac muscle is a third main type, which is also involuntary but is striated. The fibres are branched and continuous with each other. This type composes most of the heart and is confined to that organ.

Nervous Tissue

Nervous tissue is composed essentially of nerve-cells, or neurons, imbedded in supporting material. Each neuron typically has a cell-body, some short receptive processes (dendrites), and one longer, emissive process, the axon or nerve-fibre. Neurons differ greatly in

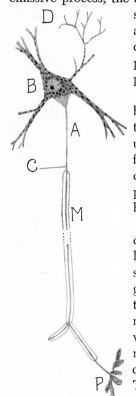

structural details as well as in size, in shape, and in the length and thickness of their processes. The nerve-fibres may or may not be provided with white myelin sheaths of a peculiar fatty substance.

A peripheral nerve is composed of parallel bundles of the microscopic nerve-fibres held together by sheaths of white connective tissue, usually with no nerve-cell bodies, though a few may be scattered along the nerve in certain places. Swellings upon the nerves at particular points are accumulations of cell-bodies and are known as ganglia.

In the brain and in the spinal cord also the cell-bodies tend to be assembled in more or less definite masses which, on account of their smaller content of myelinated fibres, have a greyer colour than the rest of the nervous tissue and are consequently known as grey matter. Elsewhere the fibres preponderate very largely, and the myelin sheaths of the myelinated fibres give such regions a whiter colour, so that the tissue is called white matter.

Fig. 7. Diagram of a typical neuron. A, axon; B, cell-body; C, collateral; D, dendrites; M, myelin sheath; P, motor end-plate.

Thus white matter is concerned mainly with simple conduction of nervous impulses and it is in grey matter that most of the connections between neurons are situated.

The neurons are imbedded in a supporting mass of tissue derived embryologically from the same source (the outermost embryonic layer) but taking no part in nervous functions. This material is the neuroglia. Through the nervous organs there run also strands of ordinary connective tissue constituting a supporting and protective framework and carrying blood-vessels, though quantitatively these form only a small part of the brain or spinal cord.

BLOOD AND LYMPH

Blood is the liquid medium for transportation through the body of oxygen, carbon dioxide, digested and absorbed food materials, waste products of metabolism besides carbon dioxide, hormones from endocrine organs, etc. Most of these are carried in solution in the intercellular liquid, the plasma, but oxygen is transported in reversible union with a red pigment, haemoglobin, which in vertebrates is confined within cell-bodies. Cells containing haemoglobin are the erythrocytes or red blood corpuscles. In mammals these have the form of biconcave discs and when mature usually lack nuclei. Very much less numerous are the leucocytes or white blood corpuscles, which are of several different kinds. Most of the leucocytes are actively motile, amoeboid cells which act as scavengers (phagocytes). They are capable of pushing through the walls of the smallest blood-vessels (capillaries) and escaping into the surrounding tissues.

In most tissues, and particularly in the connective tissues, there is a certain amount of tissue-fluid in the intercellular matrix. This is partly secreted by the cells and is supplemented by leakage of plasma and leucocytes from the blood-vessels. It is collected by minute vessels which terminate blindly in the tissue-spaces and which take in the tissue-fluid through their walls. These vessels are the lymphatic capillaries and the liquid within them is lymph.

The lymph passes through lymph glands which serve both as strainers for foreign material and as sources of new lymph cells. It is then conveyed through lymphatic vessels, which ultimately empty it into the superior caval veins. The lymphatic vessels are so thin-walled that they can not usually be observed in dissection unless specially injected with coloured materials.

CHAPTER II

ANATOMICAL TERMINOLOGY

BEFORE the description of the animal body or directions for its study can be commenced, it is necessary to have a vocabulary adequate for precise description and understood similarly by all those using it. Actually, there has grown up an exceedingly voluminous and complex terminology, which is obscured by the use of many synonyms and by the not infrequent application of the same term in two or more different ways. No attempt will be made in the present work to explain synonymy and the effort will be made to keep the special terminology to the minimum requisite for the study in hand.

Terms used are of various kinds, which may be designated general (such as artery, nerve, etc.), specific (names of particular parts), regional (e.g. abdominal, thoracic), and terms of orientation. Only the last of these need be discussed at this time, others being defined when necessary.

To begin with, the quadrupedal animal is to be imagined as standing with its body straightened out and in a horizontal position, with the limbs also straight and vertical, though hand and foot may be flat on the ground.

The upper surface of the body now is *dorsal,* the lower surface is *ventral,* and changes in position will not alter the application of these terms to the parts so defined. The sides of the body are *lateral.* An imaginary vertical plane dividing the body into right and left sides is the *median plane* and the location of anything in that plane is *median.* Anything relatively near to but not in the median plane is *medial* in contrast to the situation of anything nearer the sides of the body, which is *lateral.*

When the animal is standing in the conventional position designated, it is facing in an *anterior* direction and the opposite direction is *posterior.*

Human anatomists, however, have adopted as the conventional "anatomical position" the upright attitude of man, in which the ventral surface faces forward, and have called that surface anterior and the dorsal surface posterior. To avoid this ambiguity, the terms

11

anterior and posterior will be used as little as possible in the following account and when they are used for description the sense will be in application to a quadruped. Only in certain *names* derived from human anatomy will they unavoidably be retained as there applied. Where convenient, the term anterior will usually be replaced by *cephalic* or *cranial* and the term posterior by *caudal*. The human terms *superior* (nearer to the head) and *inferior* (further from the head) may be avoided in most but not all cases. Students should note that their reference is purely to location and has no implication of relative size or importance.

In any projecting part, such as a limb, the basal or attached end is *proximal* and the unattached end is *distal*. The same terms may be applied to arteries, nerves, etc. in a corresponding way, the connection with a larger, central or basal structure being proximal. The surfaces of a limb are described by the terms applied to the body above, though the bending of the limbs in life sometimes tends to obscure the relations. The upper surface of the hand when flat on the ground is dorsal, the lower surface volar or palmar in the fore limb, volar or planter in the hind limb.

Most of the foregoing terms, which signify *location,* may be changed to signifiy *direction* by changing the final syllable to—*ad* (e.g. *mediad, cephalad*). They may also be changed from adjectives to adverbs by adding –*ly* (e.g. *medially*).

There is also extensive use of such ordinary and self-explanatory terms as the opposed pairs: *central* and *peripheral, deep* and *superficial, internal* and *external*. The last pair, however, is sometimes used as equivalent to medial and lateral. It may be noted that *middle* (in contrast with median and its derivatives) is used for any part between two others, such as the middle finger.

Finally, the foregoing terms may be combined when appropriate. For instance a position in the more cephalic part of the dorsal region is *cephalodorsal,* a direction towards the tail and towards the ventral surface is *caudoventrad,* and so on. Even an orientation lengthwise between head and tail may be called *cephalocaudal,* or a vertical one *dorsoventral.*

Chapter III

ZOOLOGICAL POSITION

THE rabbit is a member of the great class of air-breathing, warm-blooded animals known as *Mammalia,* which class is of special interest to man since he himself belongs to it. Perhaps the most obvious and distinctive of the characteristics of this class are the possession of mammary glands and the possession of true hair.

Among the many orders composing the Mammalia, two of the more lowly are distinguished by various features related to gnawing habits, particularly modifications of the teeth for this purpose. These are the Lagomorpha and the Rodentia, formerly grouped as one under the latter name but now considered not to be very closely related. The rabbits and hares and their relatives are the *Lagomorpha,* which differ from the Rodentia most obviously in having a second pair of small incisor teeth behind the principal ones in the upper jaw, but also in many other features. Within this order the rabbits and hares constitute the family *Leporidae,* and the specific name for the European rabbit, which is that ordinarily raised in captivity and most frequently used for dissection, is *Oryctolagus cuniculus.* Upon this animal the following account is based.

Chapter IV

SKELETON—GENERAL

The skeleton constitutes the supporting system of the body, the more or less rigid framework about which the soft parts are disposed and by which in some cases they are given mechanical protection. It also serves for the attachment of muscles which move the parts of the body. Obviously, since the component materials of the skeleton are relatively rigid, they must be formed into separate pieces some, at least, of which are movably connected, otherwise any movement of the animal would be impossible. The separate pieces are usually designated, according to the material composing them, as either *bones* or *cartilages,* their connections being *articulations.*

Articulations may be nearly or quite immovable (synarthroses) or may be movable (diarthroses), the term *joint* being commonly, though not invariably, restricted to the movable connections.

The main types of relatively immovable articulation are ligamentous union (*syndesmosis*), illustrated in the bones of the wrist; *suture* (a special case of syndesmosis in which the bones have irregular, interlocking edges, as in the dorsal part of the skull); cartilage union (*synchondrosis*), exemplified between the basal bones of the skull; and attachment by fibrocartilage (*symphysis*), as between the two coxal bones of the pelvic girdle. There may also be union by continuous bony tissue (*synostosis*), producing actual fusion of two bones, as between the distal parts of the leg bones of a rabbit.

In a movable joint the surfaces of contact are so shaped as to permit smooth movement and when the joint is between bones these surfaces are covered with thin layers of cartilage to decrease friction. The two bones are held together by a sheet of ligament completely surrounding the surfaces of contact and constituting the *capsule* of the joint. This encloses a *joint cavity,* the walls of which are lined by a thin *synovial membrane* that produces a viscid liquid, *synovia,* for lubrication.

14

Movable joints are classified according to the range of move-ments permitted, which is determined by the shapes of the hard parts and by the ligaments which hold them in place. A ball-and-socket joint, or *enarthrosis* (exemplified at the shoulder), allows for movement in various directions. A hinge-joint, or *ginglymus* (as at the elbow), permits movement practically in only a single plane. A gliding joint, or *arthrodia* (as between the articular processes of the vertebrae), provides limited movement by the slipping of one surface over the other.

The internal skeleton of a vertebrate, formed by the articulation of many separate parts, as just described, consists of three basic subdivisions designated axial, visceral, and appendicular. The visceral subdivision, however, has become so reduced and so inti-mately associated with the axial subdivision in mammals that it is easier to recognize in them only the *axial* and the *appendicular* portions. The axial skeleton then comprises the vertebral column, with the ribs and the sternum, and all the skeletal parts in the head and neck. The appendicular skeleton is the hard structures in the limbs, with the basal portions, inside the body, to which these are articulated. known as the limb girdles. It may be pointed out that the appendicular skeletons of vertebrates show an extreme range of variations adapted to the habits of their possessors.

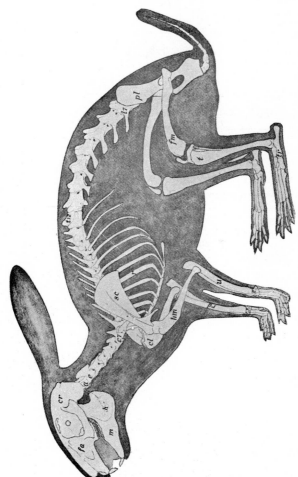

FIG. 8. Lateral view of the skeleton. From *Bensley's Practical Anatomy of the Rabbit.* a, atlas; c, carpus; c7, seventh cervical vertebra; cl, clavicle (the bone is shown above its designation); cr, cranial portion of skull; e, epistropheus; f, fibula; fa, facial portion of skull; fm, femur; h, hyoid; hm, humerus; 17, seventh lumbar vertebra; m, mandible; pl, pelvis (coxal bone); r, fifth rib; rd, radius; t, tibia; t12, twelfth thoracic vertebra; tr, tarsus.

A

THE vertebral column fo.   f the neck, trunk,
and tail regions, occupying   eld in the embryo
by a long, flexible rod, the   placement of this
flexible rod by the stronger tis   ater by still harder
bone, necessitated the moulding   into separate, articulated masses so that the body snould not become disadvantageously
rigid. Hence the vertebral column consists of a row of separate
units, *vertebrae.*

In the most primitive condition the vertebrae were all alike. The
support of the body by the limbs in a relatively non-buoyant medium
(air), however, has led to a regional differentiation in the vertebral
column of terrestrial vertebrates. Such differentiation reaches its
most extreme expression in mammals, where cervical, thoracic,
lumbar, sacral, and caudal regions are recognized. Despite the
differences in these regions, however, certain common features
remain and make it possible to describe a typical vertebra.

1. *Typical vertebra*

The vertebra consists primarily of a relatively massive basal
portion, the *centrum* or *body of the vertebra,* with an arch dorsal
to it, the *vertebral arch.* The large opening surrounded by the arch
is the *vertebral foramen* and the canal formed by these foramina in
the series of vertebrae is the *vertebral canal,* which accommodates
the spinal cord.

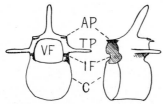

FIG. 9. Diagrams of cephalic and lateral views of a typical vertebra. AP,
superior articular process; C, centrum; IF, intervertebral foramen; TP, transverse process; VF, vertebral foramen.

17

The centrum has a shape more or less approaching cylindrical.

At each side, the vertical portion of the arch has notches in its cephalic and caudal margins so that when the vertebrae are fitted together apertures remain between them. Through these *intervertebral foramina* the spinal nerves pass.

Various projections may be added to this simple plan. There is typically a dorsal median *spinous process* and at each side there is usually a *transverse process,* these serving for muscular attachment. A pair of smaller *articular processes* on the cephalic margin of the arch and a corresponding pair on the caudal margin are present, the caudal pair overlapping the pair on the cephalic margin of the next vertebra behind. These articular processes thus form a gliding joint between adjacent vertebrae and the connection between two successive vertebrae is at three points—the articular processes and the flattened ends of the centra.

2. *Cervical region*

The seven vertebrae in this region are adapted specially for the support of the head while at the same time allowing great mobility of that part. Hence the cervical region forms a curve concave dorsally. Stretched like the string across a bow, a strong, median *dorsal ligament of the neck* is attached to the skull in front and to the thoracic vertebrae behind, but only weakly to the cervical vertebrae. Hence the spinous processes of these are only low, inconspicuous ridges. (It should be realized that the dorsal ligament of the neck is a local enlargement of a continuous ligament connecting the spinous processes of the whole series of vertebrae.) There is a distinct transverse process at each side, pierced by a longitudinal canal, the *costotransverse foramen,* so that it is attached to the side of the vertebra by two roots. The costotransverse foramen accommodates the vertebral artery as it runs forward towards the brain. All except the first two cervical vertebrae have the transverse process again divided distally into two, the ventral projection representing a reduced and fused rib.

The first cervical vertebra, or *atlas,* differs markedly from all others, its centrum having become detached during development and fused with that of the second vertebra. In consequence, the atlas has the shape of two arches set base to base, the ventral slightly smaller than the dorsal. The ventral arch accommodates a median projection (the odontoid process) from the second vertebra so that the atlas may turn on this as on a pivot. A thickened lateral mass at each side, where the bases of the two arches meet, bears a smooth *inferior articular facet,* also for articulation with the body of the second vertebra, and, facing the skull, a larger, more concave, *superior articular pit* for reception of the occipital condyle of the skull. The articulation of the skull at this point provides for nodding movement. The transverse processes are broad and flat. In front of the costotransverse foramen a groove connects it with a second opening (*oblique foramen*) which pierces the dorsal arch and conducts the vertebral artery inwards to the brain.

The second vertebra, the *axis* or *epistropheus*, is also greatly modified. In contrast with other cervical vertebrae, its form is high and rather narrow. The cephalic end of the massive centrum projects as the *odontoid process,* which in origin is the displaced centrum of the atlas. An articular facet on this process and a larger *superior articular facet* at each side of it connect with the atlas and allow the pivoting movement of the head. The articulation with the third vertebra is essentially like that between succeeding ones and allows for bending of the head sideways without twisting.

3. *Thoracic region*

The thoracic vertebrae are typically twelve in number (the presence of thirteen being a not very rare anomaly) and are characterized by their association with large, fully-developed ribs. Each of the first ten ribs has its end (head) articulated with the centra of two vertebrae, half with the one to which it belongs and half with the one in front. Hence each of the first nine thoracic vertebrae has a small *costal demifacet* on the side of the centrum at its cephalic end and another at its caudal end. The last two ribs articulate only with their own vertebrae.

The first ten thoracic vertebrae also have a second articular surface for the corresponding rib on the short, straight transverse process of each.

The spinous processes are enlarged for the attachment of the dorsal ligament of the neck. They increase in length to the third and then gradually decrease again. The first ten have a marked slant caudad.

The most caudally situated thoracic vertebrae have in addition a pair of dorsolateral *mammillary processes* rising from the superior articular processes and serving for attachment of longitudinal muscles of the back. All have the articular surfaces described for a typical vertebra, these being so placed as to permit bending of the vertebral column mainly from side to side.

4. *Lumbar region*

The seven lumbar vertebrae are larger and more massive than those so far considered, partly for support and partly for attachment of muscles used in galloping. Thus not only are the centra large but the processes for muscular attachment (spinous, mammillary, transverse) are long and strong. All the processes named have more or less slant cephalad. There is also a pair of caudolateral *accessory processes* directed caudad.

The ribs, though present in the embryo, have disappeared and are represented by the tips of the long transverse processes.

The facets on the articular processes are so placed as to permit up-and-down movement in the median plane but little sideways bending. This is just the opposite of the provision for movement in the cervical and thoracic regions.

5. *Sacral region*

The sacral vertebrae are four in number and their most distinctive feature is their fusion into a single piece, the *sacrum,* though the fusion between the fourth and third is less than that between the other vertebrae of the group. This fusion provides a firm basis for attachment of the pelvic girdle and so of the hind limb.

The first sacral vertebra is large with broad transverse processes rigidly articulated with the ilium of the pelvic girdle. (Embryologically a reduced remnant of a rib is present between these but it is indistinguishable in the mature structure.) The other vertebrae decrease successively in size and in the development of their processes.

6. *Caudal* or *coccygeal region*

The caudal vertebrae are usually sixteen. All are small, the third the largest. The tail lacking powerful muscles, there are no prominent processes for muscular attachment. The first seven vertebrae have vertebral arches to accommodate the filum terminale and the caudal spinal nerves, the rest are only solid rods of bone (centra).

7. *Ribs*

The ribs are appendages of the vertebrae. Traces of them occur along nearly the whole column but they are distinct in the adult only in the thoracic region. Normally there are twelve pairs.

Each rib includes a dorsal *costal bone* or *bone rib* and a shorter, ventral, *costal cartilage.*

The bone rib has a rounded end, the *head,* which articulates with the centrum of the corresponding thoracic vertebra and also with the posterior part of the centrum in front. The head is connected by a slightly narrower *neck* to the *body* of the rib, at the beginning of which is a projection, the *costal tubercle.* The tubercle of each of the first ten ribs articulates with the transverse process of the vertebra and each from second to eighth has a sharp dorsal projection for attachment of muscular slips.

The costal cartilage forms with the ventral end of the bone rib an angle which is acute in the first rib and becomes increasingly obtuse caudad. The first seven costal cartilages articulate with the sternum and the ribs of which they form part are called *true* or *sternal ribs* the remaining five being designated *false.* The ventral ends of the last three cartilages lie freely in the soft tissues and these ribs are consequently designated *floating ribs.* (The eighth rib is attached to the seventh and the ninth to the eighth.)

The oblique position of the ribs should be noted in a mounted skeleton since this position is essential for the breathing movements described on page 75.

8. *Sternum*

The sternum or breast bone is a median ventral rod in the thoracic region, composed of six distinct segments, the *sternebrae.* The most cephalic segment is named the *manubrium sterni,* the most caudal the *xiphoid process.* The last has a broad, thin plate of cartilage at its free tip in the rabbit.

The clavicle (part of the pectoral girdle) is connected to the anterior end of the manubrium by ligament and the first seven costal cartilages articulate directly with the sternum.

B. SKULL

1. The skull is the main supporting framework of the head and also encloses and protects the brain and the internal ear. The latter functions are performed by the *cranial portion* and in front of this projects the more purely supporting *facial portion,* which includes the jaws and is long and narrow in the rabbit. The elongated jaws are associated with feeding habits in which almost sole dependence is placed upon them with little or no direct assistance from the limbs and, in this case, are associated particularly with the gnawing habit.

The skull is composed of many distinct bones and a few cartilages, all of which components except the mandible and the ossicles of the middle ear are immovably articulated with their neighbours.

In the embryo the brain-case develops as a trough of cartilage, open dorsally, with capsules for the internal ears and the nasal organs included in its walls. This is known as the chondrocranium.

Later, centres of ossification appear and transform most of the cartilage into a series of replacing bones. At the same time plate-like membrane bones form a roof over the brain and supports for the face and jaws. The membrane bones and the replacing bones soon become completely incorporated together so that it is impossible to distinguish them without knowledge of their developmental history. The sutures become gradually less conspicuous but in the rabbit most of them remain clearly visible even in old specimens.

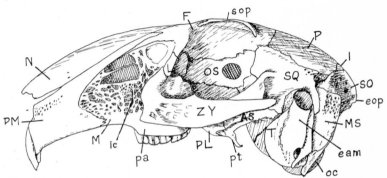

Fig. 10. Lateral view of the skull. AS, alisphenoid bone; F, frontal bone; I, interparietal bone; L, lacrimal bone; M, maxilla; MS, mastoid portion of the petromastoid bone; N, nasal bone; OS, orbitosphenoid bone; P, parietal bone; PL, palatine bone; PM, premaxilla; SO, supraoccipital bone; SQ, squamosal bone; T, tympanic bone; ZY, zygomatic bone; eam, external auditory meatus; eop, external occipital protuberance; ic, cephalic opening of infraorbital canal; oc, occipital condyle; pa, alveolar process of maxilla; pt, pterygoid process (medial lamina) of alisphenoid; sop, supraorbital process.

2. Laterally, the cranial and facial portions of the skull are partly separated by the deep, rounded, *orbital cavity,* which in the intact animal lodges the eye and various associated structures. This is bridged externally by a long, bony *zygomatic arch.*

3. Caudally, the cranial portion of the skull has a broad, roughly flat surface, the *nuchal surface,* which faces the neck and is approximately perpendicular to the floor and roof of the brain-case and to the axis of the first few cervical vertebrae. This surface is formed entirely by the *occipital bone,* a composite structure produced by the developmental fusion of a *supraoccipital bone,* paired lateral *exoccipital bones,* and a median ventral *basioccipital bone.* Between these it is pierced by a large, median *foramen magnum,* through which the brain connects with the spinal cord. At each side of this a smooth prominence, the *occipital condyle,* functions for articulation with the atlas.

The nuchal surface is separated from the dorsal surface by a sharp ridge, which has a prominent median projection, the *external occipital protuberance.* The dorsal ligament of the neck is attached to this to support some of the weight of the head.

4. The dorsal surface of the skull is markedly curved. In front of the supraoccipital is a small, median *interparietal bone* separating the supraoccipital from a pair of *parietal bones* which make up much of the roof of the brain-case. In front of these again the pair of large, irregular *frontal bones* not only completes this roof but also bears prominent supraorbital processes and extends ventrad in the walls of the orbits. Anterior to the frontals, a pair of long, narrow *nasal bones* roofs the nasal cavities.

5. In lateral view the exoccipital bone is nearly concealed by a bone shaped somewhat like an inverted cone and distinguished by its pitted surface. This is the *mastoid portion* of the *petromastoid bone,* the bone which encloses the internal ear. The other part, the *petrous portion,* of this bone is completely concealed by the mastoid portion and by the prominent, round, inflated-looking *tympanic bulla* in front of it. The bulla is formed by the tympanic bone and contains the middle ear. Dorsally the bulla continues into a short, wide, bony tube with a large opening which in the natural condition would be continued into the aperture of the external ear. This whole tube is the *external acoustic meatus.*

Dorsal and anterior to the parts just mentioned, the lateral wall of the brain-case is formed largely by the *squamosal bone,* a plate of very irregular outline with a prominent projection (*zygomatic process*) forming the caudal end of the zygomatic arch. The ventral side of the zygomatic process is hollowed out as the *mandibular fossa,* in which the elongate head of the mandible fits in a manner permitting movement backwards and forwards but not from side to side. Dorsal to the base of the zygomatic process is a groove which expands into a shallow depression, the temporal fossa, on the side of the cranium. It accommodates the temporal muscle, one of the muscles of mastication, which is smaller in the rabbit than in many mammals.

In front of the squamosal, the *alisphenoid* and *orbitosphenoid bones* appear as plates in the wall of the orbit, the orbitosphenoid being the more anterior and being distinguished by the large round *optic foramen* piercing it. A series of other openings, or foramina, none quite so large as the optic, extends along the cranial wall between lateral and ventral surfaces and serves for ingress and egress of the cranial nerves and blood-vessels.

The cephalic wall of the orbit is formed ventrally by the *maxilla,* which here appears as a prominent ridge containing the roots of the molar teeth, and more dorsally by a thin, loosely-articulated plate, the *lacrimal bone,* the lateral margin of which projects beyond the rim of the orbit.

The *maxilla* is a large bone extending forward from the region where it has just been observed and forming an extensive portion of the facial region. A prominent *zygomatic process* constitutes the anterior root of the zygomatic arch and is fused with the anterior end of the *zygomatic* (or *jugal*) *bone,* which forms the main portion of the arch. Ventral and caudal to the base of the zygomatic process, a massive portion of the bone (*alveolar process*) contains the roots of the cheek teeth. In front of these processes the maxilla has a markedly spongy structure in the rabbit. An infraorbital canal through the base of the zygomatic process transmits nerves and vessels between the orbit and the face.

The premaxilla forms the most anterior part of the upper jaw, being articulated with its fellow of the other side in the median plane and with the maxilla caudally. In it are inserted the roots of the incisor teeth. It also bounds the anterior part of the nasal cavity ventrally and laterally. A long, slender, *frontal process* extends dorsocaudad along the lateral margin of the nasal bone.

6. In ventral view the three median elements composing the floor of the brain-case may be observed, namely, the basioccipital, the basisphenoid, and the presphenoid bones. The *basioccipital,* the most caudal, is fused at each side with the exoccipital bones and extends forward between the tympanic bullae. It is joined by a conspicuous synchondrosis to the wedge-shaped *basisphenoid* in front of it. About the middle of the basisphenoid there is a circular foramen opening into the interior of the bone. At each side the basisphenoid is continuous dorsolaterally with the alisphenoid, which has already been observed from a lateral viewpoint and which extends ventrally as the *pterygoid process* for the attachment of muscles of the jaw. Each pterygoid process consists of diverging *medial* and *lateral laminae.* Another synchondrosis in front of the basisphenoid connects it with the *presphenoid,* which is visible only as a narrow strip at the bottom of a deep, narrow, median depression. The presphenoid is fused at each side with the orbitosphenoid, but this connection is completely concealed in the intact skull by the palatine bone.

The paired *palatine bone* appears as a prominent, thick, ventral ridge or plate at the side of the deep median depression mentioned above (in which the nasopharynx is situated). Its caudal end is notched and articulates with the two laminae of the pterygoid

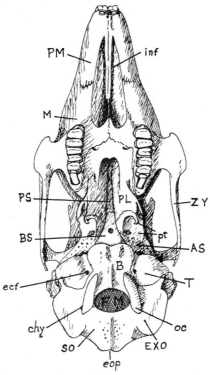

Fig. 11. Ventral view of the skull. AS, alisphenoid bone; B, basioccipital bone; BS, basisphenoid bone; EXO, exoccipital bone; FM, foramen magnum; M, maxilla; PL, palatine bone; PM, premaxilla; PS, presphenoid bone; SO, supraoccipital bone; T, tympanic bone; ZY, zygomatic bone. chy, external opening of hypoglossal canal; ecf, external carotid foramen; eop, external occipital protruberance; inf, incisive foramen; oc, occipital condyle; pt, pterygoid process of the alisphenoid.

process. It extends dorsad as a thinner plate, part of the lateral surface of which is exposed in the wall of the orbit. Passing forward medial to the alveolar process of the maxilla, it articulates with that bone and spreads mediad to meet its fellow of the other side, thereby constituting the caudal portion of the *hard palate*, which separates oral and nasal cavities. Caudal to this a low longitudinal ridge runs along the medial surface of the palatine bone towards the pterygoid process and marks the line of attachment of the soft palate.

In front of the palatine bone the hard palate is continued by the ventral portions of the maxilla and the premaxilla. In the rabbit these are pierced by a pair of long, narrow, *incisive foramina,* continuous across the median line in their caudal third. The foramina open to the nasal fossae.

7. By looking into the external nasal apertures, it is possible to see delicate, scroll-like, bony folds within, though these can not be studied in detail without opening the nasal fossae. In life they are covered by nasal epithelium. The more posterior part of this is olfactory, the more anterior merely warms (and may moisten) the air and helps to free it from foreign particles.

8. The ventral portions of the nasal fossae are separated by a median, curved, vertical plate of bone, the *vomer.* It is partly visible through the incisive foramina but can be adequately observed only in a divided skull.

9. The *mandible* is composed of paired bones united by a symphysis in the rabbit. The horizontal part of the two constitutes the *body of the mandible* and the posterior, vertical part of each is the *ramus.* The lower teeth are borne by the body.

The ramus projects ventrocaudally as the *angle of the mandible.* Dorsally it bears the long, narrow, articular surface on a slightly thickened *head.* Separated from the head by a small notch, the anterodorsal margin of the ramus has a low, curved ridge, the *coronoid process,* on which the temporal muscle is inserted. The lateral surface of the ramus has a broad, shallow depression occupied by the insertion of the masseter muscle. The medial surface of the ramus has a pronounced depression in its dorsal part for insertion of the superior portion of the external pterygoid muscle and ventral to this is covered by the insertion of the internal pterygoid. Just in front of these insertions a vertical slit in the medial surface of the bone, the *mandibular foramen,* permits the passage of nerves and blood-vessels to the interior of the mandible and to the lower teeth. A continuation of the nerve emerges on the lateral surface through the *mental foramen* to serve the region of the chin.

10. *Teeth* are borne in sockets by the mandible, by the maxilla, and by the premaxilla. At the anterior end of each jaw are sharp, chisel-like *incisor* teeth. These are followed by a long gap at each side, the *diastema,* and canine teeth, which occur in this region in a

more typical mammalian dentition, are absent. Behind the diastema occur the *cheek teeth,* divided into *premolars* and *molars,* distinguished by the fact that premolars are present in both first and second sets of teeth, molars only in the second set.

The numbers of these different kinds of teeth in the rabbit may be represented by the *dental formula*: i $\frac{2}{1}$, c $\frac{0}{0}$, pm $\frac{3}{2}$, m $\frac{3}{3}$. This gives the number of each kind on one side in each of upper and lower jaw.

The incisor teeth are of the rodent type. These are permanently growing teeth with a layer of enamel on the anterior surface only. The rest of the tooth, being composed of dentine, wears away more quickly than the harder enamel so that a sharp cutting edge of enamel is maintained by the gnawing habits of the animal. There is a single pair of incisors in the mandible but each premaxilla has one large incisor and a second, smaller or accessory one set in behind the first.

The cheek teeth of the rabbit have flattened ends with prominent ridges of enamel disposed transversely. Thus the ridges are approximately at right angles to the principal direction of movement of the jaw in chewing and constitute an efficient grinding surface.

11. The *hyoid apparatus* is derived from embryonic visceral arches and functions as a support for the tongue, in the base of which it is imbedded, lying between the angles of the mandible. It includes a median *hyoid bone* and two pairs of rod-shaped structures the *greater* and *lesser cornua,* articulated with the lateral edges of this bone. These cornua do not articulate directly with the skull but are connected with the jugular process of the occipital bone by muscles, respectively the stylohyoideus major and the stylohyoideus minor.

The cartilages of the larynx and trachea, which are described with the soft parts (p. 94), also are derived from the visceral skeleton.

Chapter VI

SKELETON–APPENDICULAR SUBDIVISION

A. Anterior Limb

1. The *pectoral girdle,* that portion of the skeleton of the anterior limb which is imbedded in the trunk of the animal, comprises two pairs of bones, the *clavicles,* or collar bones, and the *scapulae,* or shoulder blades. It is attached to the axial skeleton only by ligaments and muscles, without direct articulation, so that the shock when the animal lands suddenly on its fore feet is taken up by these elastic structures.

The *clavicle* is particularly small and slender in the rabbit, about the size of a common pin, and is suspended by ligaments between the shoulder and the cephalic tip of the sternum.

The *scapula* is an approximately triangular plate lying against the side of the thorax so that its surfaces are medial and lateral. The three edges are directed roughly, one towards the head (superior border), one towards the vertebral column (vertebral border), and one towards the arm-pit (axillary border). The cephalo-ventral angle is thickened and bears a smoothly-rounded *glenoid cavity,* into which fits the head of the humerus. This cavity is partly overhung by a short but prominent projection mediad, the *coracoid process,* which is a vestige of a separate coracoid bone, one of the three primary elements of the pectoral girdle. A conspicuous longitudinal ridge, the *scapular spine,* divides the lateral surface into supraspinous and infraspinous fossae, which are filled in the intact animal by muscles originating from their surfaces and serving to move the humerus. The spine projects anteroventrally as the *acromion* (terminal) and the *metacromion* (at right angles to the axis of the spine) and provides insertion for muscles moving the shoulder. The slight depression occupying the whole medial surface of the scapula is the *subscapular fossa,* which also serves for muscular origin. In the fresh condition a narrow, tapering plate of cartilage, the suprascapula, runs along the vertebral border.

2. The *humerus* is the support of the upper arm and is a typical long bone consisting of a shaft, or diaphysis, with an epiphysis at each end. These three parts are developed by separate centres of ossification within the primary, cartilaginous humerus of the embryo.

The proximal end has a smooth, rounded, swollen *head* which fits into the glenoid cavity of the scapula, and, in front of the head, roughened *greater* (lateral) and *lesser* (medial) *tubercles* for muscular insertion. From the greater tubercle an elongate, roughened area, the *deltoid tuberosity,* also for the attachment of muscles, extends along the cephalolateral surface of the bone for more than a third of its length.

At its distal end the humerus has a pulley-like articular surface, the *trochlea,* which fits against radius and ulna. Rough areas just proximal to the articular surfaces are the *medial* and *lateral epicondyles* for the origin of muscles of the forearm.

3. The radius and ulna are the bones of the forearm. Both are long, slender, and somewhat curved and the radius crosses the ulna from a position cephalodorsal to it at the proximal end to a medial position at the distal end. The proximal ends of both bones enter into the formation of a deep, crescentic, *semilunar notch,* into which fits the trochlea of the humerus. Proximal to this notch the ulna projects prominently as the *olecranon,* which bears the insertions of the extensor muscles for the elbow-joint and provides leverage for their action.

The radius and ulna have flattened surfaces of contact at their proximal and distal ends and are held closely together by an *interosseous ligament* so that no movement between them is possible and rotation of the forearm can not occur as it does in man.

A conspicuous epiphysis at the distal end of each bone articulates with the proximal wrist bones.

4. The *carpus,* or wrist, is composed of nine small carpal bones. The arrangement of these is slightly modified from the fundamental

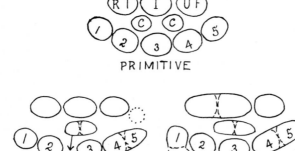

PRIMITIVE

RABBIT CARPUS   RABBIT TARSUS

Fig. 12. Diagrams of left carpal and tarsal bones. C, central bones; I, intermedium; RT, radiale or tibiale; UF, ulnare or fibulare.

pattern of the wrist and ankle of terrestrial vertebrates, which involved three proximal bones, one or more central bones, and five distal bones. (Fig. 12).

In the rabbit the three proximal carpal bones remain and are named mediolaterad, *navicular, lunate,* and *triquetral.* The central bone has been displaced into the distal row and the two most lateral distal carpals have fused into one bone called the hamate. The elements appearing in the distal row are named mediolaterad, *greater multangular, lesser multangular, central, capitate,* and *hamate.*

An additional bone, not represented in the primary plan but formed in the tendon of one of the muscles (flexor carpi ulnaris), occurs ventral to the triquetral and is named *pisiform.*

5. The *metacarpus* includes five small, long bones articulating with the distal carpals and supporting the region corresponding with the palm of the hand. The first is markedly reduced.

The *phalanges* are the bones of the fingers, the most proximal in each articulating with the corresponding metacarpal and the most distal being curved and tapered to fit into the sheath-like claw. The first digit has two phalanges, each of the other digits three.

6. *Sesamoid bones* are accessory elements, usually small, developed in the tendons of muscles (thus coming into the classification as membrane bones). The pisiform bone mentioned above is one of these and smaller ones occur at some of the joints of the hand.

B. Posterior Limb

1. The *pelvic girdle* differs from the pectoral in being directly articulated to the vertebral column so as to provide for the transmission to the body of the powerful thrust of the hind limbs in locomotion as well as for simple support. In adaptation to the forward direction of this thrust, the girdle is elongate and its originally dorsal part (the ilium) extends almost straight forward from the articulation of the thigh to the attachment to the sacrum.

The girdle is composed of a pair of *coxal bones* united in the midventral line by a symphysis. This symphysis, commonly termed pubic from its relations in man, is better called the *pelvic symphysis* since it involves both pubis and ischium in the rabbit and other quadrupeds. Each coxal bone is made up of three primary components fused so completely in the adult that the lines of union are not usually visible.

The dorsal component is the *ilium,* which extends cephalad from the *acetabulum,* the depression which receives the head of the femur.

Its basal part is thick and narrow but it expands into a broad *iliac wing* for articulation with the sacrum and for the origin of muscles of the hip.

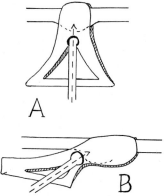

Fig. 13. Diagrams of right lateral view of the pelvis; A, in a quadruped where the weight of the body bears mainly straight down on the hind legs; B, in a quadruped where the chief force from the hind legs is in a thrust cephalad (as in the rabbit).

Behind the acetabulum, the line of the ilium is directly continued by the *ischium*, originally the caudoventral component of the coxa, which terminates in a roughened and thickened *ischial tuberosity*. The dorsal margin of the bone bears a short, sharp *ischial spine*, which functions for muscular origin and divides the margin into two long, smooth, shallow depressions, the *lesser sciatic notch* behind the spine and the *greater sciatic notch* in front of it (about half of the greater notch formed by the ilium). The ischium is bifurcated, a thinner ventral portion extending cephalomediad to enter into the constitution of the symphysis and to fuse with the third main component of the coxa, the pubis. Its posterior margin forms an acute angle or nearly a right angle with that of the other side.

The *pubis* is the cephaloventral component of the coxa and in-cludes a longitudinal branch, united at the symphysis with the corresponding part on the opposite side, and a nearly transverse branch extending from the symphysis to the acetabulum. Enclosed between the pubis and the ischium is a large opening, the obturator foramen, which has muscles attached all round its margin and provides room for their transverse swelling when they contract in action.

The *acetabulum* is a deep, circular cup for articulation with the head of the femur at the point where the ilium, the ischium, and the pubis meet. In the rabbit, however, the pubis is shut out from the articulation by a small accessory bone, the *os acetabuli*. A rough depression at the bottom of the cup and a notch in its side provide attachment for a strong ligament (round ligament of the femur) holding the femur in place.

2. The *femur*, or thigh bone, is long, strong, and slightly curved. At the proximal end, a nearly hemispherical *head* for articulation projects somewhat mediad on a stout, constricted *neck*. Beside this are two prominent, roughened projections for the insertion of muscles, the *great trochanter* proximal and lateral, the *lesser trochanter* medial.

Distally a pair of smooth eminences, the *medial* and *lateral condyles*, articulate with the tibia and roughened areas, *medial* and *lateral epicondyles*, serve for muscular attachment on the sides of the bone. A broad, shallow depression, the *patellar surface*, permits the knee-cap (patella) to slide along it in the natural condition.

3. The *tibia* and *fibula*, the two parallel long bones of the leg, are completely fused distally in the rabbit for somewhat more than half their length, though proximally there is a space between them except at the very end. This space is occupied by a sheet of ligament. The tibia is thick and strong, the fibula slender. The proximal end has slightly concave surfaces on *medial* and *lateral condyles* fitting against the corresponding condyles of the femur and on the front of the bone a sharp, longitudinal ridge, the *tibial tuberosity*, bears the attachment of the patellar ligament, through which the extensor muscles of the thigh are inserted. The distal extremity of the combined bone has articular surfaces for the two proximal bones of the ankle, the talus and the calcaneus.

4. The *tarsus*, or ankle, is based on a fundamental pattern identical with that of the wrist but is more modified than is the wrist (Fig. 12).

The proximal row of tarsal bones has its two more medial elements fused as the *talus*, a bone bearing a large, pulley-like eminence, the *trochlea tali*, for articulation with the tibia, this being the most important part of the ankle joint. The lateral proximal tarsal, the *calcaneus*, is greatly enlarged. It has a raised articular surface for the fibular side of the tibiofibula and a long, heavy projection, the *tuber calcanei*, which forms the heel.

Distal to the talus, the roughly rectangular *navicular* represents the central bone of the basic pattern.

The distal row of tarsals, like the distal carpals, has the fourth and fifth elements fused, producing a bone known as the *cuboid*.

The three more medial elements are named *first, second,* and *third cuneiform bones* respectively but, since the first digit is lost in the rabbit, the first cuneiform is fused with the second metatarsal and only the second and third remain distinct.

5. The first *metatarsal bone* is reduced to an inconspicuous splinter ventral to the base of the second and the navicular. The second, third, fourth, and fifth, however, are long and strong, giving leverage in leaping.

Each developed metatarsal bears the proximal unit of a row of three *phalanges.* The distal phalanx in each case is tapered to fit into the claw, just as in the digits of the anterior limb.

6. *Sesamoid bones* occur in various joints, much the largest and most prominent being the *patella,* or *knee-cap,* which is situated in the insertion-tendon of the extensor muscles of the thigh where it passes over the end of the femur. Three other sesamoids are found in the origin-portions of muscles of the calf where they might be pinched by the bending knee.

Chapter VII

EXTERNAL FEATURES

THE outer surface of the body of a mammal has a characteristic covering of *hairs,* which are secondary outgrowths of the epidermis, the outer layer of the skin. This coat of hair is very complete in the rabbit, being absent only over the eyes and in a pair of depressions beside the external genital organs, the inguinal spaces.

The organism may be regarded as comprising *head, neck, trunk, limbs,* and *tail.*

In the head there is an anterior *mouth* bounded by upper and lower lips, with a pair of nostrils dorsal to it, the external openings being connected by deep grooves so that the upper lip is divided. On the anterior, or *facial* region a few hairs are greatly enlarged and act as tactile organs, the *vibrissae.* In the more posterior, or *cranial* region of the head the *eyes* are very prominent, each guarded by upper and lower eyelids with a third eyelid in the anterior angle between the other two. The eyes are directed more nearly laterad than in other mammals. Behind them are long *external ears.*

The anterior limb is articulated to the body at the shoulder and comprises *upper arm, forearm,* and *hand,* the last having five *digits* each with a long, curved claw. Between the upper arm and trunk is a depression, the *axillary fossa.*

The posterior limb likewise comprises three main divisions, the *thigh,* the *leg,* and the *foot,* and is separated from the trunk by the *inguinal furrow.* Only four digits are fully developed in the rabbit.

The trunk includes the *thorax,* enclosed by the ribs, the *abdomen,* which lacks such protection, and the *back,* or *dorsum,* containing the vertebral column and the mass of large muscles associated with it. Ventral to the base of the tail, the trunk is penetrated by the external opening of the digestive system, the *anus.* Deep hairless depressions, the inguinal spaces, lie beside it. Just ventral to the anus in the female is the *vulva,* the opening of the urinogenital passage surrounded by folds of skin, with the tip of a small, flexible rod, the *clitoris,* in its ventral wall. In the corresponding position the male has the *penis,* a projecting organ with its tip pierced by

34

the urinogenital aperture and surrounded by a free fold of skin, the *prepuce.* At each side of the penis is a sac, the *scrotal sac,* containing the essential reproductive gland, the *testis.*

Various parts of the skeleton can be recognized by feeling. Among these there should be identified the *angle of the mandible* at the posteroventral part of that organ and the *symphysis* where the two halves of the mandible are united anteriorly, the *manubrium sterni* at the cephalic end of the sternum, the *xiphoid process* at the posterior end of the sternum, the *iliac crest* at the anterodorsal extremity of the pelvic girdle, to which the hind limb is attached, and the *pubic* or *pelvic symphysis* by which the two halves of this girdle are united ventrally.

CHAPTER VIII

MUSCLES OF THE LIMBS

WITHIN the body the soft parts are to various degrees supported and protected by the skeleton, which has already been described. This framework of rigid parts has to be moved by muscles in order that locomotion and other activities of the animal may take place. Hence an examination of internal parts may reasonably begin with representatives of the muscular system. Further, the slender limbs are subject to desiccation if the dissection is extended over a prolonged period so that there is some advantage in completing their study before the trunk is opened.

In all dissection of muscles the main points to be observed, besides the shape, size, and position of each, are the *origin*, the *insertion*, and the *direction* of the fibres. The origin is the relatively immovable point of attachment, the insertion the relatively movable point which is pulled towards the origin when the muscle contracts. Hence the precise determination of these three characters makes it possible to recognize the *action* of the muscle, it being kept in mind that a muscle can act only by contraction, pulling but never pushing.

The action of a muscle as determined by the examination indicated in the previous paragraph is, however, a somewhat theoretical abstraction, most movements in the living animal being performed by delicately coordinated groups of muscles and involving both synergic and antagonistic groups. Thus the effect produced by any one muscle acting in the living body may be modified from moment to moment by the activities of many others simultaneously excited.

The muscles of the limbs are mostly capable of being classified according to whether they bend (*flex*) or straighten (*extend*) the limb. Besides flexor and extensor muscles, however, *rotators*, which twist the limb on its own axis, *abductors*, which move the limb away from the median plane, and *adductors*, which move it towards the median plane, are also recognized.

In the application of the terms flexor and extensor, it is necessary to imagine the limb as originally projecting straight out from the side of the horizontal body with the palm of the hand and the sole

36

of the foot facing the ground. Any muscle which bends the limb down towards the ground may then be termed flexor and any which bends it up extensor. These relations are retained despite the changes which have taken place in the relative positions of the parts of the limbs. Thus the muscles which bend the foot upwards at the ankle are still termed extensors and those which straighten the ankle are termed flexors.

In dissection the points of attachment stated for each muscle should be identified first on cleaned bones and then precisely located by feeling in the specimen. Any fascia or other obscuring tissue should be neatly removed so that the muscle running between the points of attachment is clearly visible and the muscle should be completely freed from all other structures except at the points of functional attachment named (origin and insertion). Also nerves and blood-vessels entering the muscle should be preserved as far as possible. When a muscle has been studied and must be divided to expose parts below, it should be cut right through approximately half way between its origin and its insertion and in a direction roughly at right angles to its fibres. Its halves may then be reflected, or folded back, while still attached to origin and insertion so that the relations may be checked and re-examined as the dissection proceeds.

A. ANTERIOR LIMB

To start dissection of the anterior limb, the skin should be cut through in the median ventral line of the body from about the xiphoid process forward to about the level of the angle of the mandible. A transverse incision from the caudal end of the median cut should extend round on one side just behind the shoulder to the dorsal median line and a second should pass from the anterior end of the median cut just behind the ear on the same side. A further incision should sever the skin along the medial surface of the anterior limb to the elbow and should there completely encircle the limb. The flap of skin thus outlined should now be lifted at the median incision and torn gently away from the underlying muscles, to which it is attached by loose, spongy, white *subcutaneous connective tissue*. The end of a finger or a blunt instrument may be used to assist in tearing the skin free, but cutting should be avoided if possible. In this way the skin must be worked free from the upper arm and from the side of the chest and neck and folded back to the mid-dorsal line. The skin of the forearm and hand should be removed later, when dissection of these parts is to be commenced.

An exceedingly thin sheet of muscle, the *platysma,* often removed with the skin, covers the neck just under the latter. It is continuous from side to side dorsally and continuous caudally with a somewhat thicker sheet, the *cutaneous maximus muscle,* over the trunk. Beneath the platysma, a more definite band extends from the manubrium sterni to the base of the external ear, the *depressor conchae posterior.* If still in place, these muscles and surrounding connective tissue should be removed. The large *external jugular vein* should be noted running along the ventrolateral aspect of the neck.

If a briefer dissection, omitting the muscles of the shoulder, is desired, the skin may be cut only round the proximal end and along the medial or the lateral surface of the upper arm and may then be removed from upper arm and forearm by tearing the subcutaneous connective tissue as described above.

1. *Muscles which pull the pectoral girdle towards the axial skeleton*

(a) *Cleidomastoideus.* Originates on the mastoid process of the skull and is inserted on the middle of the clavicle. Its action depends upon whether other muscles are holding the head or the clavicle more rigidly in place.

(b) *Basioclavicularis.* Originates on the basioccipital bone and is inserted on the lateral third of the clavicle and on the ligament attaching this to the limb.

(c) *Levator scapulae major.* Has its origin just in front of the preceding, on the basioccipital bone at its articulation with the basisphenoid. The insertion is on the tip of the metacromion.

(d) *Trapezius.* In the rabbit this muscle has two portions narrowly continuous at their origins. The *superior portion* originates on the external occipital protuberance of the skull and the dorsal ligament of the neck (the median ligament attaching the skull to the spinous processes of the thoracic vertebrae). The insertion is on the metacromion and the fascia over the muscles in the supraspinous fossa of the scapula. The origin of the *inferior portion* continues from that of the superior along the series of tips of spinous processes of the thoracic vertebrae to the lumbodorsal fascia, a thick sheet of white connective tissue covering the back. (The skin on the trunk and the thin underlying cutaneous maximus muscle should be loosened and raised sufficiently to reveal this origin of the trapezius.) The insertion of the inferior portion is on the caudal side of the dorsal half of the scapular spine. The ventral edge of the inferior portion is more or less fused with another muscle, the latissimus dorsi, to be described later.

The basioclavicularis, the levator scapulae major, and both portions of the trapezius should be divided so that the scapula may be pulled laterad and the next four muscles may be examined.

(*e*) *Rhomboideus minor.* The origin is on the dorsal ligament of the neck and the insertion on the vertebral border of the scapula.

(*f*) *Rhomboideus major.* The origin is on the first seven (or more) thoracic spinous processes and the insertion on the caudal third of the vertebral border of the scapula.

Division of the two rhomboideus muscles facilitates examination of the next. The latissimus dorsi—2(*a*) below—may also be divided.

(*g*) *Levator scapulae minor.* A narrow band originating on the back part of the skull and extending across the medial aspect of the scapula to be inserted at the inferior angle.

(*h*) *Serratus anterior.* Represented by two separate portions. The *cervical portion* has its origin on the transverse processes of the last five cervical vertebrae and on the first two ribs, its insertion on the medial edge of the vertebral border of the scapula. The *thoracic portion* rises by a series of separate slips from a variable series of ribs, usually the third to the ninth, these slips converging to be inserted on the vertebral border of the scapula. If the limb is held firmly, the thoracic portion may serve to raise the ribs in forced breathing.

2. *Muscles which pull the humerus towards the axial skeleton (and, in part, the pectoral girdle)*

(*a*) *Latissimus dorsi.* This muscle originates in the lumbodorsal fascia and on the last four ribs, its dorsal edge covered by and more or less fused with the inferior portion of the trapezius. It passes medial to the humerus to be inserted on the deltoid tuberosity.

(*b*) *Pectoralis primus.* A distinct band with origin on the manubrium sterni and insertion (concealed by another muscle not yet described, the cleidohumeralis) on the deltoid tuberosity. It should be freed from the larger muscle beneath it and divided.

The remaining pectoral muscles are so closely associated and so easily split almost anywhere, by reason of their loose texture, that there is disagreement as to how many should be recognized. The points of attachment must be identified with particular care to ensure separating the muscles as described.

(*c*) *Pectoralis secundus.* The largest pectoral muscle, this originates on the ventrolateral aspect of the sternum throughout its length and is inserted on the proximal two-thirds of the anterior surface of the humerus. Starting at the clavicle, the muscle should be carefully separated from those it covers and should be divided.

(*d*) Dorsal to the pectoralis secundus lie the pectoralis tertius (subdivided) and the pectoscapularis, dorsal to it, these crossing the shoulder to be inserted together on the spine and superior border of the scapula. The pectoralis quartus, inserted on the humerus, lies just caudal to the p. tertius.

3. *Blood-vessels and nerves in the axillary fossa*

The remaining pectoral muscles and the clavicle should now be divided, after which step the blood-vessels and nerves may be completely cleared of any obscuring connective tissue. Axillary lymph-glands may be noted in this tissue.

(*a*) Arteries

The blood-supply of the limb reaches it almost entirely through the *axillary artery*. This is the direct continuation of the vessel known as the subclavian artery before it reaches the axillary fossa, and its name is again changed, to brachial artery, when it leaves the fossa.

The first branch of the axillary artery is the *transverse scapular artery*, which runs over the shoulder to the supraspinatus muscle.

Next the *thoracoacromial artery* runs between pectorales tertius and quartus and supplies pectoral muscles, platysma, and skin.

Arising close to or usually in common with the thoracoacromial, the *lateral thoracic artery* passes caudad, supplying the pectoralis secundus and continuing into the abdominal wall.

The *subscapular artery* supplies the muscle (subscapularis) on the medial surface of the scapula and continues along the dorso-lateral aspect of the trunk.

Near where it enters the arm as the brachial, the axillary artery gives off circumflex and deep arteries which pass into the proximal end of the arm.

(*b*)Veins

The axillary vein lies close and somewhat caudal to the corresponding artery. It is the continuation across the axillary fossa of the cephalic vein of the arm (p. 46) and receives tributaries accompanying the arterial branches. Medially it continues as the subclavian vein.

(*c*) Nerves

The nerves in the axillary fossa connect with the last five cervical and the first thoracic spinal nerves. They are linked by numerous and variable connecting strands to form a network, the *brachial plexus*. This is probably due to the developmental history, which involves the rearrangement in the limb muscles of material derived from several embryonic segments. As each part of this material is supplied by nerve fibres from its own segmental nerve, the plexus results.

Three principal nerves from the plexus enter the limb, the *radial, median,* and *ulnar,* the distal course of which will be indicated below. Proximally these connect chiefly with a stout trunk formed by union of the ventral branches of the eighth cervical and the first thoracic nerves.

Two *subscapular nerves* supply the teres major and the subscapular muscles respectively, a branch runs to the latissimus dorsi, and one (*suprascapular nerve*) passes round the front of the scapula to the supraspinatus muscle. (The muscles mentioned are described in the next section.)

All parts still attaching the limb to the body should now be divided.

4. *Muscles which pull the humerus towards the pectoral girdle so as either to extend, to flex, or to rotate the shoulder joint*

Before these are separated, the *cephalic vein* should be noted. This superficial vessel comes from the anterodorsal surface of the forearm and runs up the anterior surface of the arm, then crosses its lateral aspect and turns mediad to reach the axillary fossa after receiving tributaries from the muscles about the shoulder.

(*a*) *Cleidohumeralis.* This muscle has its origin on the lateral portion of the clavicle and on the connecting ligament so that it appears as a direct continuation of the basioclavicularis, which is inserted where this originates. Its insertion is on the distal part of the anterior surface of the humerus.

(*b*) *Deltoideus.* The triangular *acromial portion* originates on the acromion and is inserted on the distal part of the deltoid tuberosity of the humerus. The *scapular portion* originates on the infraspinous fascia (the thick connective tissue surrounding the muscle in the infraspinous fossa of the scapula) a short distance from the vertebral border. It passes under the metacromion, on which additional fibres take origin, and tapers into a thin tendon under the acromial portion, with which it is inserted.

The scapular portion must be carefully separated from the muscle which it covers, the infraspinatus, and must be divided and reflected, the metacromion being broken through to permit this.

(*c*) *Infraspinatus.* Filling the infraspinous fossa of the scapula, this muscle has its origin on all parts of the bone in the fossa. Its insertion is on the greater tubercle of the humerus.

(*d*) *Supraspinatus.* The insertion portions of the pectoralis tertius and the pectoscapularis must be removed to reveal this muscle. It occupies completely the supraspinous fossa of the scapula and originates on the whole surface of this fossa and on the superior border of the bone. The insertion is on the greater tubercle of the humerus.

(*e*) *Subscapularis.* This muscle takes origin from the whole medial surface of the scapula and corresponds rather closely with its outlines. The insertion is on the lesser tubercle of the humerus.

(*f*) *Teres major.* The origin is on the dorsal portion of the axillary border of the scapula and the insertion the anterior surface of the humerus, in common with the latissimus dorsi.

(*g*) *Teres minor.* This is a very small muscle concealed between the ventral part of the infraspinatus (with which it is closely associated) and the teres major. If the infraspinatus is pressed away from the lateral aspect of the teres major and the thick tendon of origin of the long head of the triceps (which is described with the next group), the slender teres minor may be seen. It originates on the more ventral portion of the axillary border of the scapula and crosses the lateral surface of the tendon mentioned to be inserted on the greater tubercle. It is thus an antagonist of the much larger teres major in rotatory movements of the humerus.

(*h*) *Coracobrachialis.* The origin is the coracoid process, the insertion the medial surface of the humerus about one-third of its length distally.

5. *Muscles which bend or straighten the elbow joint*

A. Extensors (lying mainly behind the axis of the humerus).

(*a*) *Extensor antibrachii parvus.* A thin muscle with its origin in the middle of the fascia on the medial aspect of the arm, its insertion on the medial surface of the olecranon. The fascia should be severed and the muscle folded back.

(*b*) *Anconaeus minimus.* A very small, thin, almost square muscle having its origin on the medial epicondyle of the humerus and its insertion on the medial surface of the olecranon, where it is covered by the previous one.

(*c*) *Triceps brachii.* The three heads referred to in the name are practically separate muscles with a common insertion on the olecranon. The long head has its origin on the ventral part of the axillary border of the scapula, the lateral head on the greater tubercle and adjoining surface of the humerus, the medial head on practically the whole posterior surface of the humerus.

B. Flexors (lying mainly in front of the humerus)

(d) *Biceps brachii*. Only one of the two heads referred to in the name is present in the rabbit. It originates by a tendon attached to the cephalic edge of the glenoid cavity of the scapula and is inserted by another tendon on the medial surface of the radius and on the ventromedial surface of the ulna only a short distance distal to the articulation with the humerus.

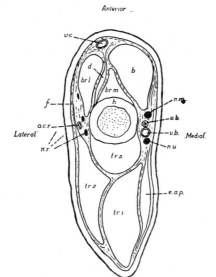

Fig. 14. Diagram of transverse section through the distal portion of the arm. From *Bensley's Practical Anatomy of the Rabbit*. ab, brachial artery; acr, radial collateral artery; b, biceps muscle; brl and brm, lateral and medial heads of the brachialis; d, deltoideus (insertion portion); eap, extensor antibrachii parvus; f, brachial fascia; h, humerus; nm, median nerve; nr, radial nerve; nu, ulnar nerve; tr1, tr2, tr3, long lateral, and medial heads of the triceps; vb, brachial vein; vc, cephalic vein.

(e) *Brachialis*. Originating on the anterior and lateral surfaces of the humerus and inserted in common with the biceps, the proximal end is divided into a larger lateral and a smaller medial portion by tendons of insertion of the pectoralis secundus and cleidohumeralis muscles.

6. *Muscles which move the wrist and the digits*

A. Extensors

The long, slender tendons of insertion are distributed to the dorsal aspects of the digits, mostly after passing under a *dorsal carpal ligament* which holds them together just proximal to the joint of the wrist. The origins are mainly lateral or anterodorsal and the muscles are bound together by very firm fascia, which must be dissected away. It is easiest to identify the tendons of insertion first and then trace them in a proximal direction.

(*a*) *Extensor carpi radialis longus.* Originates on the lateral epicondyle of the humerus and is inserted on the proximal end of the second metacarpal.

(*b*) *Extensor carpi radialis brevis.* This also originates on the lateral epicondyle and is partly fused with the preceding. The insertion is on the proximal end of the third metacarpal.

(*c*) *Abductor pollicis.* Originating on the anterolateral surfaces of the radius and ulna and inserted on the proximal end of the first metacarpal, the abductor pollicis has a rather thick tendon which forms a cross with the associated tendons of the two previous muscles.

(*d*) *Extensor pollicis et indicis.* The origin of this also is on the anterolateral surfaces of the radius and ulna but the slender tendon of insertion is the most medial of a group of five passing under the dorsal carpal ligament and divides to be attached to the ungual phalanx of the first digit and to the distal end of the second metacarpal.

(*e*) *Extensor digitorum communis.* Originates on the lateral epicondyle of the humerus and the adjoining part of the ulna and is inserted by four separate tendons which pass together under the dorsal carpal ligament and are attached to all the phalanges of the second to the fifth digits.

(*f*) *Extensor digiti quarti proprius.* Originates on the lateral epicondyle and is inserted by a long slender tendon on the ungual phalanx of the fourth digit.

(*g*) *Extensor digiti quinti proprius.* Originates close to the preceding on the lateral epicondyle and is inserted in the fifth digit on the distal end of the metacarpal and the proximal end of the first phalanx.

(*h*) *Extensor carpi ulnaris.* Originates on the lateral epicondyle and on the proximal part of the ulna and is inserted at the proximal end of the fifth metacarpal.

B. Flexors.

The origins are in general medial, in contrast to those of the extensors, and the insertions are on the volar surface. The tendons of insertion are held together at the wrist by a strong *transverse carpal ligament*, which should be cut.

(*a*) *Pronator teres.* The origin is on the medial epicondyle of the humerus and the insertion on the ventral surface of the radius, the muscle not reaching the wrist.

(*b*) *Flexor carpi radialis.* This also originates on the medial epicondyle but is inserted by a long tendon on the proximal end of the second metacarpal.

(*c*) *Flexor digitorum sublimis.* The origin is partly on the medial epicondyle (in common with the ulnar part of the flexor digitorum profundus) and partly on the adjacent region of the ulna. The insertion is on the second phalanges of the second to the fifth digits.

(*d*) *Flexor carpi ulnaris.* Originates on the medial epicondyle and on the medial surface of the olecranon and is inserted by a stout tendon on the pisiform bone.

(*e*) *Palmaris.* Between the foregoing and the first head of the following muscle, the palmaris is very small. It has its origin on the medial epicondyle, its insertion by a very slender tendon on the fascia of the palm.

(*f*) *Flexor digitorum profundus.* Originates in four parts or heads; the *superficial* on the medial epicondyle, the *ulnar* on the medial epicondyle, the *radial* on the ventral surface of the radius, and the *middle* portion on the ventral surface of the ulna. After uniting distally these give rise to five tendons which perforate those of the flexor sublimis at the metacarpo-phalangeal joints to be inserted at the proximal ends of the ungual phalanges of the five digits.

7. *Muscles which move only individual digits*

These are very small muscles originating in the region of the wrist or on the metacarpals.

(*a*) *Flexor digiti quinti.*

(*b*) *Lumbricales.*

(*c*) *Adductor digiti quinti, adductor digiti quarti, adductor indicis.*

(*d*) *Flexor pollicis brevis.*

(*e*) *Interossei.*

8. *Blood-vessels and nerves in the anterior limb*

(*a*) Arteries

The blood-supply of the limb is obtained through the *brachial artery*, a direct continuation of the axillary. The brachial artery passes along the medial side of the upper arm, giving off various branches. Upon reaching the medial surface of the radius it divides into the median artery and the ulnar artery. Branches of these are distributed to all the more distal parts of the limb.

(b) Veins

The *brachial vein* accompanies the brachial artery and its chief tributaries correspond with the branches of the latter.

The *cephalic vein* is a superficial vessel on the anterodorsal surface of the forearm. It passes up the lateral surface of the arm and joins the brachial vein to form the axillary vessel.

(c) Nerves

The *radial nerve*, originating in the axillary fossa as a derivative of the brachial plexus, runs behind the brachial artery to the posterior surface of the humerus. Distally it divides into a superficial branch to the dorsum of the hand and a deep branch to the extensor muscles of the forearm.

The *median nerve* runs from the brachial plexus in front of the brachial artery and accompanies the latter to the forearm, passing then with the median artery to the palm of the hand.

The *ulnar nerve* passes round the medial surface of the elbow, accompanies the ulnar artery through the forearm, and is distributed to the palm of the hand.

B. Posterior Limb

If time is available for dissection of both limbs, an instructive comparison between the main groups of muscles may be made in the light of the different orientation of the limb-segments. For study of the posterior limb the skin should be divided along the medial surface of the thigh and cut round the leg just below the knee, then stripped off as far as the mid-dorsal line. The distal parts should be uncovered later, when the dissector is ready to examine them.

As in the anterior limb, the muscles are to be considered in functionally related groups.

1. *Muscles which pull the proximal end of the hind limb forward, bending the back*

Examination of these must be deferred until the abdominal viscera have been removed. At the present stage the dissector must proceed to the second group of muscles.

(a) *Psoas minor.* The origin is on the ventral surfaces of the last four lumbar vertebrae. The insertion is on the anterior margin of the pubis by a tendon which crosses a flat ligamentous band extending from the middle of the inguinal ligament to the ventral surface of the first sacral vertebra. (The inguinal ligament is a strong white cord stretched between the anterior end of the pelvic symphysis and the iliac crest.)

The tendon of insertion and the inguinal ligament must be divided.

(*b*) *Psoas major.* Originates on the bodies of the last three thoracic vertebrae, with their ribs, and on those of all the lumbar vertebrae and is inserted on the lesser trochanter of the femur.

(*c*) *Iliacus.* The origin is on the last lumbar and first sacral vertebrae and the insertion on the lesser trochanter.

(*d*) *Quadratus lumborum.* Dorsal to the psoas major, the lateral edge of which should be pulled ventromediad. The origin is on the bodies of the last five thoracic vertebrae and their ribs and on the bodies of all the lumbar vertebrae, the insertion on the transverse processes of six lumbar vertebrae and on the ilium.

2. *Muscles which extend or abduct the limb at the hip*

As a preliminary to examination of the first of these, the first portion of the biceps (p. 50) should be divided, as follows. Find the sciatic vein on the dorsolateral surface of the thigh and cut through the fascia close to its proximal portion, about half an inch in length. From here a line in the fascia is usually obvious running distad and towards the knee. Continuation of the incision along this line will free the first portion of the biceps from the muscles behind it. Another line in the fascia is visible in a transverse position between the sacrum and the tip of the great trochanter, whence it extends along the lateral aspect of the thigh. A cut along this line to meet the first incision will free the first portion of the biceps, which can now be divided and folded back.

(*a*) *Glutaeus maximus.* The origin is in two portions joined by a sheet of thickened fascia, or aponeurosis, one from the fascia dorsal to the sacrum, the second from the anteroventral edge of the wing of the ilium, where it is continuous with the origins of two other muscles (tensor fasciae latae and first head of the rectus femoris) to be described later. The insertion is on the third trochanter of the femur.

Both parts of the muscle must be divided to expose the next.

(*b*) *Glutaeus medius.* The origin is largely from the anterior edge of the ilium and extends to the fascia over the first two sacral vertebrae. The insertion is on the great trochanter and in the trochanteric fossa.

Division of this muscle exposes the next.

(c) *Glutaeus minimus*. This originates from the entire lateral surface of the ilium and is inserted on the great trochanter.

(d) *Tensor fasciae latae*. With its origin on the anteroventral edge of the ilium and its insertion in the thick fascia (the fascia lata) on the lateral aspect of the thigh, this muscle is completely fused with that in front of it (first head of the rectus femoris) and largely with that behind (second part of the glutaeus maximus).

(e) *Piriformis*. This originates on the second and third sacral vertebrae and is inserted on the first trochanter, passing through the greater sciatic notch.

(f) *Gemellus superior*. The origin is on the ischial spine and just in front of it, the insertion, by a thick tendon shared with the next two muscles, on the lateral wall of the trochanteric fossa.

(g) *Obturator internus*. The origin on the internal surface of the coxal bone all round and in front of the obturator foramen is not visible laterally. The conspicuous tendon of insertion passes through the lesser sciatic notch between the two gemelli and fuses with their tendons.

(h) *Gemellus inferior*. This originates on the posterior part of the ischium, including the tuberosity, and is inserted by the tendon shared with the two just described.

(i) *Quadratus femoris*. The origin is ventral to the more caudal part of the preceding, the insertion on the third trochanter and distal to it and in the trochanteric fossa.

(j) *Obturator externus*. Having its origin on the outer surface of the coxal bone round the obturator foramen and its insertion in the trochanteric fossa, this muscle can not be clearly seen until those of the next group have been examined and divided.

3. *Muscles which adduct the limb at the hip*

For study of these it is necessary first to examine and remove the sartorius and gracilis muscles (p. 50), which also adduct the limb but flex the knee in addition.

(a) *Pectineus*. This rather small muscle originates on the pecten of the pubis and is inserted on the femur just distal to the second trochanter.

(b) *Adductor brevis*. The origin is on the anterior part of the pelvic symphysis and the insertion just distal to that of the pectineus.

(c) *Adductor longus*. The origin is on the posterior part of the symphysis and the inferior ramus of the ischium, the insertion on the posterior surface of the femur.

(*d*) *Adductor magnus.* Originates on the ventral surface of the ischium, mainly on the tuberosity, and is inserted on the mediodistal part of the femur, spreading on to the tibia.

4. *Muscles acting on the knee-joint*

A. Extensors

These together constitute the *quadriceps femoris.* They have a common insertion on the tuberosity of the tibia by a stout tendon in which a large sesamoid bone, the patella, is developed. The portion of the tendon between the patella and the tibia is known as the *patellar ligament.*

(*a*) *Rectus femoris.* In the rabbit this appears as two distinct muscles. The first part is superficial and has its origin on the iliac

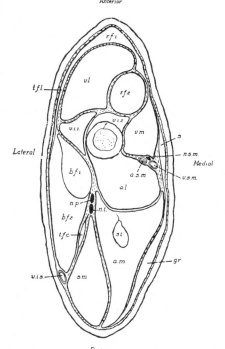

Fig. 15. Diagram of transverse section through the middle of the thigh. From *Bensley's Practical Anatomy of the Rabbit,* al. adductor longus muscle; am, adductor magnus; asm, femoral artery; bf1 and bf2, first and second heads of the biceps femoris; f, femur; gr, gracilis; np, peroneal nerve; nsm, greater saphenous nerve; nt, tibial nerve:, rf1 and rf2, first and second heads of the rectus femoris; s, sartorius; sm, semimembranosus; st, semitendinosus; tfc, tensor fasciae cruris; tfl, tensor fasciae latae; vil and vi2, first and second heads of the vastus intermedius; vis, sciatic vein; vl, vastus lateralis; vm, vastus medialis; vsm, great saphenous vein.

wing, fused with the tensor fasciae latae. The second part is concealed from the surface and is cylindrical in form, its origin being by a stout tendon from the inferior anterior spine of the ilium.

Both parts should be divided.

(b) *Vastus lateralis.* This, the largest of the group, originates on the great trochanter and the thick fascia lateral to it.

(c) *Vastus intermedius.* Two distinct parts are described under this name, the first originating on the third trochanter and lying just behind the vastus lateralis, the second originating along the anterior surface of the femur.

(d) *Vastus medialis.* The origin is on the medial surface of the neck of the femur and the muscle lies just behind the rectus femoris.

B. Flexors

Lying behind the femur so as to be antagonistic to the foregoing, their insertion portions enclosing the popliteal fossa, these are sometimes known as the hamstring muscles.

(a) *Sartorius.* A very slender band originating on the inguinal ligament and inserted, fused with the gracilis, medial to the proximal end of the tibia, this muscle acting alone would be mainly a rotator.

(b) *Gracilis.* A thin sheet originating along the pelvic symphysis and inserted in the fascia of the proximomedial surface of the leg.

The sartorius and the gracilis must be divided if that has not already been done.

(c) *Biceps femoris.* The two heads from which the muscle is named are quite separate. The first (already divided—p. 47) has a broad origin over the last three sacral and first three caudal vertebrae and a narrow insertion on the lateral edge of the patella. The second head has a narrow origin on the ischial tuberosity and a broad insertion on the fascia of the lateral surface of the leg.

(d) *Tensor fasciae cruris.* This very slender muscle lying under the biceps originates from the fourth sacral vertebra and is inserted on the lateral fascia of the leg.

(e) *Semimembranosus.* This thick muscle bifurcates proximally, originating partly in the superficial fascia over the first head of the biceps and, more largely, deep to the biceps, on the lateral process of the ischial tuberosity. It is inserted with the gracilis in the proximal medial fascia of the leg (whence a tendinous band continues distad into the tendon of the heel).

(f) *Semitendinosus.* Its origin on the ischial tuberosity and its insertion on the medial condyle of the tibia, this is completely enclosed by the adductor magnus and may be observed by splitting the latter.

5. *Muscles which move the foot at the ankle*

A. Extensors

Lying in front of the leg and inserted on the dorsum of the foot, these muscles bend the foot upwards.

(*a*) *Extensor hallucis longus.* The origin is on the anteromedial surface of the tibia. The tendon of insertion passes under the medial malleolus and reaches the dorsal surface of the proximal phalanx of the second (first functional) digit.

(*b*) *Tibialis anterior.* The origin is on the lateral condyle and the tuberosity of the tibia. The insertion is by a long tendon which passes under an oblique *crural ligament* near the distal end of the leg and reaches the base of the second metatarsal bone.

The muscle may be divided.

(*c*) *Extensor digitorum longus.* A stout tendon of origin is attached to the lateral edge of the patellar surface of the femur and traverses the knee joint. The muscle proper underlies the tibialis

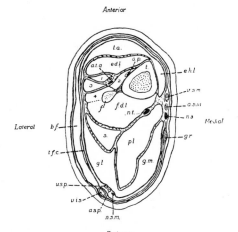

Fig. 16. Diagram of transverse section of the proximal portion of the leg. From *Bensley's Practical Anatomy of the Rabbit.* asm, great saphenous artery; asp, small saphenous artery; ap, ata, anterior tibial artery; bf, biceps femoris (insertion portion); edl, extensor digitorum longus; ehl, extensor hallucis longus; f, fibula; fdl, flexor digitorum longus; gl and gn, lateral and medial heads of the gastrocnemius; gr, gracilis (tendon of insertion); ns, greater saphenous nerve; nsm, lesser saphenous nerve; nt, tibial nerve; pl, plantaris; s, soleus; t, tibia; ta, tibialis anterior; tfc, tensor fasciae cruris (insertion); vis, sciatic vein; vsm, great saphenous vein; vsp, small saphenous vein; 1-4, peroneus longus, brevis, tertius and quartus.

anterior on the anterolateral aspect of the leg. The insertion tendon runs under the crural ligament and under a *cruciate ligament* on the dorsal surface of the foot before dividing into four parts which are attached to all phalanges of the respective digits.

B. Peronaeus group

Though the muscles of this group individually may function as flexors or extensors, their main action is that of lateral tractors or abductors. Their slender fleshy portions are partly fused proximally and their long, thin tendons of insertion run together through a deep groove (peroneal notch) posterior and lateral to the lateral malleolus of the tibiofibula. They are retained in the groove by a ligament (retinaculum peronaeum), which should be cut so as to free them.

(*a*) *Peronaeus longus.* The origin is on the lateral condyle of the tibia and the head of the fibula, the insertion on the reduced first metatarsal, the tendon crossing the plantar surface of the cuboid bone.

(*b*) *Peronaeus brevis.* The origin is on the lateral condyle and the shaft of the tibia, the insertion on the lateral tubercle at the proximal end of the fifth metatarsal.

(*c*) *Peronaeus tertius.* Originates on the head of the fibula and the adjacent interosseous ligament, the muscle being fused with the flexor digitorum longus. The insertion is on the fifth metatarsal and its phalanges.

(*d*) *Peronaeus quartus.* The origin is similar to that of the peronaeus tertius and the insertion is on the fourth metatarsal.

C. Flexors.

Lying behind the tibiofibula, these muscles actually straighten the foot at the ankle but bend the toes.

(*a*) *Triceps surae.* The three heads for which this muscle is named have a common insertion by the *tendon of the heel* or *Achilles' tendon,* which is attached to the ventral surface of the calcaneus, under cover of the tendon of the plantaris. They are:

(1) *Lateral head of the gastrocnemius,* attached to the lateral condyles of tibia and fibula;

(2) *Medial head of the gastrocnemius,* attached mainly to the medial condyle of the femur but also to the lateral condyle and to the patella;

(3) *Soleus,* attached by a tendon to the head of the fibula.

(*b*) *Plantaris.* The origin is on the lateral condyle of the femur and the tendon of insertion passes round the heel to the plantar surface, dividing to reach the second phalanges of the four digits.

The triceps and the plantaris should be divided.

(c) *Popliteus.* A short muscle passing from the lateral condyle of the femur obliquely to the posteromedial edge of the proximal part of the tibia.

(d) *Flexor digitorum longus.* Origin is on the posterior surface of the proximal parts of the tibia and fibula. The tendon of insertion passes round the posterior end of the talus to the plantar surface, where it divides into parts for the ungual phalanges of the four digits.

6. *Muscles which move individual digits*

These are the three lumbricales, the adductores indicis et minimi digiti, and the interossei.

7. *Blood-vessels of the posterior limb*

The blood-supply is mainly through the *femoral artery,* which runs along the medial surface of the thigh giving off branches to this region. Approaching the knee, the femoral artery divides into the *great saphenous artery* to the medial surface of the leg and the *popliteal artery.* The popliteal artery passes between the tibia and the fibula to their anterior surface, giving branches to the adjacent muscles, and then divides into the *anterior tibial* and the *peroneal arteries,* both of which reach the dorsal part of the foot, the peroneal in the more lateral positon.

The proximal muscles of the thigh are also supplied in part by the *sciatic artery,* which comes from the interior of the pelvis through the greater sciatic notch and runs caudad along the ischium.

The *femoral vein* accompanies the femoral artery and receives tributaries corresponding with the branches of the latter.

The *sciatic vein* runs along the posterolateral surface of the thigh, where it has been used as a landmark in dissecting the muscles, and enters the pelvic cavity.

8. *Nerves of the posterior limb*

Two main nerves, the *femoral* and the *sciatic,* enter the limb, both derived from a network, the lumbosacral plexus, formed by the last four lumbar and the sacral spinal nerves. This can not be examined at the present stage of the dissection.

The *femoral nerve* enters the thigh beside the femoral artery and divides at once into a branch ramifying to the anterior muscles and another branch, the *great saphenous nerve,* which accompanies the femoral and great saphenous arteries.

The larger *sciatic nerve* enters the thigh through the greater sciatic notch and is exposed by division of the biceps muscle. It distributes branches to the posterior thigh-muscles and forms two main subdivisions which run close together to the knee and then diverge. These are the *peroneal nerve* in front and the *tibial* behind and their branches reach all the more distal parts of the limb.

CHAPTER IX

THE JOINTS OF THE HIP AND THE KNEE

EXAMPLES of the structure of joints may be examined most satis-
factorily in the posterior limb, where these are relatively strongly
developed.

Each articulation is enclosed in a capsule formed by a sheet of
strong connective tissue extending from one bone to the other and
completely enclosing a cavity containing the articular surfaces. Each
of these surfaces is covered by a very thin layer of cartilage and the
cavity contains a small amount of lubricating liquid, the synovia,
secreted by the lining of the capsule, the synovial membrane.

The capsules at the hip and at the knee should be exposed by
removing the muscular attachments about them as thoroughly as is
practicable.

A. THE HIP-JOINT

The articulation here is a ball-and-socket joint, the rounded head
of the femur fitting into the cup-like acetabulum, though movement
is not equally free in all directions. The enclosing capsule is attached
round the neck of the femur and to the margin of the acetabulum.
It is somewhat thickened in three regions, constituting the rather
indefinite dorsal *ischiocapsular,* anterior *iliofemoral,* and ventral
pubocapsular ligaments.

After division of the capsule the internal surfaces of the joint
are exposed and the head of the femur is seen to be attached to the
coxal bone by a thick *round ligament.*

B. THE KNEE-JOINT

The articulation in this case forms a hinge-joint, though movement is not rigidly confined to one plane. The structure is more
complex than that of the hip-joint. The capsule is attached to the
femur round the edges of the condyles and the patellar surface and
similarly to the tibia round the edges of its condyles. Outside the
capsule stout medial and lateral bands, the *tibial* and *fibular*
collateral ligaments, hold the two bones together. The capsule is
also attached to four small bones which have articular surfaces
taking part in the formation of the joint, namely the patella and

three other sesamoid bones embedded in the two heads of the gastrocnemius and in the popliteus muscles respectively. The patellar ligament forms part of the capsule and the joint is traversed by the tendons of origin of the popliteus and of the extensor digitorum longus.

Within the joint the femur and the tibia are held together by an *anterior cruciate ligament* and a *posterior cruciate ligament,* both attached to the femur in the intercondyloid fossa. Curved cushions of cartilage, the *medial* and *lateral menisci,* are inserted between the apposed condyles and are held in place by additional ligaments. The medial meniscus is attached to the tibia only but the lateral meniscus is connected to both tibia and femur, the ligament to the femur lying behind the posterior cruciate ligament.

Chapter X

ABDOMINAL WALL

For dissection of the abdominal wall the specimen should be laid upon its back and a median incision through the skin only should be made from the sternum back to the pelvic symphysis. Transverse incisions should then be made from the ends of the longitudinal one, passing just behind the shoulder and just in front of the hip. The skin can now be lifted on one side and pulled away from the underlying muscles, to which it is attached by loose *subcutaneous connective tissue,* the point of a finger or the blunt handle of a scalpel being used to help to tear the attachment. Cutting with a sharp edge should be avoided so far as possible.

The structures to be examined in this dissection are mostly muscles and, although these are spread into very thin sheets, the main points to be observed are the same as in the muscles of the limbs, namely, shape, size, position, origin, insertion, and direction of the fibres.

1. The thick, tough, inner layer of the skin is the *corium.* The loose, spongy, subcutaneous tissue under the corium contains large quantities of fat in many mammals but not usually in rabbits. It is similar to the connective tissue between and round the individual muscles, where it is known as *fascia.*

In the female the mammary glands lie in the subcutaneous layer and are connected by ducts with the mammary nipples in the skin.

2. A white line is visible in a median position extending from the xiphoid process to the pelvic symphysis. This is the *linea alba,* a cord of tendon attached to the skeleton at each end and hence able to serve for the attachment of the muscles lying at each side of it.

The remaining parts to be mentioned, lying lateral to the linea alba, are all paired.

3. A very thin sheet of muscle, the *cutaneus maximus,* covers the surface and has its origin on the linea alba, its insertion on the inner surface of the skin of the sides and back, so that it functions for shaking the skin. The fibres pass caudodorsad from their origin. This muscle should be divided and folded back to expose the next.

4. The *external oblique muscle* has its origin to a small extent on the xiphoid process but mainly from the posterior ten ribs (by

distinct, separate slips) and on the lumbodorsal fascia. The latter is a thick sheet of white connective tissue covering the back in the posterior thoracic and lumbar regions and attached to the tips of the spinous processes of the vertebrae. Some of the more anterior slips of origin are concealed by muscles of the chest.

The insertion of the external oblique muscle is on the linea alba and the inguinal ligament, the latter a stout cord extending from the iliac crest to the pelvic symphysis. The attachment to the linea alba is by a thin but strong tendinous sheet, or aponeurosis, the junction with this of the fleshy muscle proper appearing as a distinct curved line some distance lateral to the linea alba. The fibres of the external oblique muscle in general run caudoventrad.

5. The external oblique muscle should be cut along a line approximately from the posterior tip of the sternum to the crest of the ilium (both of which may be identified by feeling) and separated from the muscle beneath.

The *internal oblique muscle,* thus exposed, has its origin on the inguinal ligament, the lumbodorsal fascia, and the last four ribs, the fibres slanting cephaloventrad to join the edge of an aponeurosis wider than that of the external oblique. Through this it is inserted on the linea alba.

6. Enclosed between two layers of the semitransparent aponeurosis of the internal oblique, may be seen the *rectus abdominis muscle,* a flat longitudinal band lying close beside the linea alba. It is attached to the lateral surface of the sternum anteriorly and to the pelvic symphysis posteriorly.

7. Between the lateral edge of the rectus abdominis muscle and the aponeurotic line of the internal oblique it is usually possible to see through the aponeurosis fibres running approximately at right angles to those of the internal oblique. These are part of the *transverse abdominal muscle,* the deepest muscle of the abdominal wall, which originates on the seven last ribs, the lumbodorsal fascia, and the inguinal ligament and is inserted by a rather narrow aponeurosis on the linea alba.

8. The inner surface of the transverse muscle is covered by a thin, transparent layer of connective and epithelial tissues constituting the *parietal peritoneum.*

The oblique and transverse muscles function mainly for the support of the visceral organs. The rectus abdominis, in addition, is active in bending the body as in galloping. Also all take part in expiration (p. 75).

CHAPTER XI

DIGESTIVE SYSTEM (ABDOMINAL PORTIONS)

THE incisions through the abdominal wall should now be completed, the viscera, or organs in the abdominal cavity, being thereby exposed.

The abdominal cavity is the largest of four portions into which the primary body cavity, the coelom, has become divided, the others being the pericardial cavity, which surrounds the heart, and the two pleural cavities, which contain the lungs.

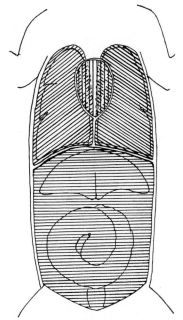

FIG. 17. Diagram representing the division of the primary coelom. Pericardial cavity hatched vertically, pleural cavities hatched obliquely, peritoneal cavity hatched horizontally.

The inner surface of the wall of the abdominal cavity is lined by the parietal peritoneum, mentioned at the end of the previous chapter. If this thin, smooth, moist layer is traced from either side

59

to the dorsal median line, it is found there to turn inward, combining with the corresponding sheet from the other side to form a free membrane extending across to the digestive tube and dividing to continue over the surface of the latter. The free sheet thus formed is the *mesentery* and the continuation over the surface of the digestive or other organ is the *visceral peritoneum*. The parietal peritoneum, the mesentery, and the visceral peritoneum are thus parts of one continuous *serous membrane*, which is not interrupted anywhere, so that it may be considered that no organs are really *within* the abdominal cavity. When the free, double sheet of peritoneum extends between two organs, as the stomach and the liver, it is called an *omentum*, or sometimes a *ligament*. When the abdomen is opened, the organs appear to be slung in their peritoneal coverings but actually the mesenteries do not give important mechanical support to the digestive organs. Rather they provide a path by which vessels and nerves may pass to and from these organs without interrupting the continuity of the serous membrane.

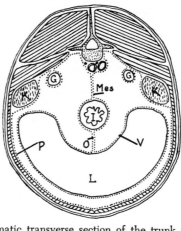

FIG. 18. Diagrammatic transverse section of the trunk region of a mammal to show the relations of the peritoneum (represented by a dotted line). G, gonad; K, kidney; I, intestine; L. liver; Mes, mesentery; O, omentum; P, parietal peritoneum; V, visceral peritoneum.

With a little caution the organs now exposed may be moved about and examined freely but *the peritoneal attachments should not be torn and the positions of the parts should not be disturbed so seriously that they cannot readily be re-determined.* Nearly all of these organs belong to the digestive system, the coiled mass of intestines being most conspicuous and the smooth, brown liver lying

in front of it. By gently pressing the intestines in a caudal direction and tipping the edge of the liver towards the head, one may examine the stomach, which lies between them.

1. The stomach has a convex caudoventral surface, the *greater curvature,* and a concave cephalodorsal surface, the *lesser curvature.* The latter is connected by a sheet of peritoneum, the *lesser omentum,* to a part of the liver. From the greater curvature, another sheet of peritoneum extends a short distance as a free, loose fold, the *greater omentum,* which often contains fat and which turns back on itself and extends dorsad to adhere to part of the intestinal mesentery (transverse mesocolon).

If the lesser omentum is torn, a narrow tube, the *oesophagus,* will be seen entering the stomach from in front.

The region of the stomach entered by the oesophagus is known as the *cardia.* To the left of it, a large bulge is the *fundus.* The right hand portion of the stomach is the *pyloric limb* and between this and the fundus and cardia is the *body of the stomach.*

A sharp constriction, the *pylorus,* marks the connection of the stomach with the intestine. Here an annular thickening of the circular muscle, the *pyloric sphincter,* acts as a valve to regulate passage of contents from the stomach.

2. From the pylorus, the *small intestine* curves round, as the *superior portion of the duodenum* (receiving the bile duct), to run caudad on the right side of the body as the *descending portion of the duodenum.* It then forms an irregular, twisted, *transverse portion* and passes towards the head again as the *ascending portion of the duodenum.* The duodenum of a rabbit thus appears as a long, U-shaped loop and, if this is turned over towards the animal's left, the ascending portion seems to end abruptly in the mesentery at a point arbitrarily considered to mark the beginning of the next division, the *mesenterial small intestine.*

The mesenterial small intestine is further subdivided into jejunum and ileum, distinguished by the thinner wall and less rich vascularity of the second portion, but the difference between these is not usually very apparent in embalmed specimens. The mesenterial small intestine is long and greatly coiled and its terminal portion is expanded in the rabbit into a rounded, very thick-walled *sacculus rotundus.*

3. The sacculus rotundus opens into the *large intestine,* which, in general, is distinguished by being wider than the small intestine, though this is not true at all points.

At the very beginning of the large intestine, there is a blind diverticulum which is absent or small in carnivores but is very large in herbivorous mammals. This is the *caecum*. In the rabbit it is markedly wider than any other part of the intestine and is so long that it is coiled in a flat spiral. Most of the caecum is very thin-walled and has a spiral constriction which marks the line of attachment of an internal fold, the *spiral valve*, but the terminal portion, the *vermiform process* or *appendix*, is narrower and has a thick wall. The vermiform process is about as large in a rabbit as it is in a man.

In contrast with the caecum, the portion of the large intestine leading on towards the anus from the opening of the sacculus rotundus is the *colon*, but in the rabbit the peculiar character of the caecum (its greater width and thinner wall) has been secondarily extended a short distance along this.

As a result of the disposition in the human body, the colon is described as comprising ascending, transverse, and descending portions. The elongation that appears in all parts of the intestine of a rabbit in adaptation to its vegetable diet is particularly marked in the ascending colon, which passes alternately cephalad and caudad so that it can be considered to consist of five "limbs", the first running towards the head, the second towards the tail, and so on. The third limb is complicated by the formation of a secondary loop towards the left side.

The area of the wall of the colon is increased and passage of contents is delayed by the formation of deep sacculations, or *haustra*.

The ascending colon ends on the right side dorsal to the pyloric limb of the stomach. It is continued by the *transverse colon*, a short, wavy division passing to the left and then turning caudad in an approximately median position as the *descending colon*.

The descending colon disappears from the abdominal cavity and is continued without any structural change through the pelvis as the short *straight intestine*, or *rectum*, which ends in the anus. The rectum will be exposed in a later dissection.

4. The abdominal portion of the digestive tube is supplied with blood by three main arteries running from the dorsal aorta through the mesentery, namely, the coeliac artery, the superior mesenteric artery, and the inferior mesenteric artery. Each of these branches to reach its distribution and the ramification of the coeliac artery may profitably be examined.

The stomach should be gently turned towards the right and the peritoneum dorsal to it should be torn with forceps, the connective tissue and fat being scraped away until the aorta and two large median arteries (and the coeliac and superior mesenteric ganglia— p. 66) become visible. The more anterior artery is the *coeliac*, the more

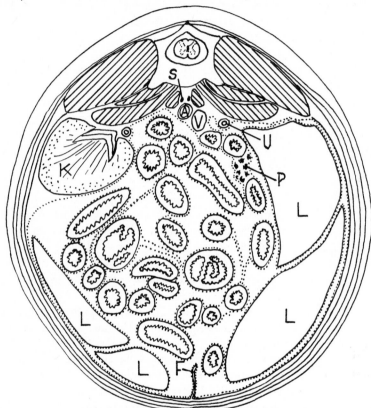

Fig. 19. Diagram of a transverse section of the trunk of a rabbit, showing the relations of the peritoneum (represented by a dotted line), for comparison with Fig. 18. A, abdominal aorta; F, middle umbilical fold; K, left kidney; L, liver; P, pancreas in mesoduodenum; S, sympathetic trunk; U, right ureter, V, inferior caval vein.

posterior the *superior mesenteric*. With forceps the peritoneum and connective tissue round the coeliac artery may be stripped away so as to expose the vessel completely and this process should be continued along each branch until the whole course of each is clear. The precise manner in which the branches originate is subject to much variation but the terminations are relatively constant and vessels are consequently named according to their endings without regard to their origins.

(a) The first branch of any considerable size from the coeliac artery is usually the *splenic artery,* which runs along the *spleen,* an elongate body lying dorsal to the left side of the stomach, and sends secondary branches into it. The splenic artery also gives a varying number of *short gastric arteries* to the greater curvature of the stomach. The last of these, distinguished as the *left gastroepiploic artery* runs round the greater curvature towards the right side. Finally, the splenic artery continues into the greater omentum.

(b) The coeliac artery next divides into the hepatic and the left gastric arteries. The *left gastric artery* is usually represented by several vessels which are distributed to both dorsal and ventral surfaces of the stomach, those to the ventral surface passing round both sides of the cardia.

(c) The *hepatic artery* gives rise to a large *gastroduodenal artery* which divides near the pylorus into branches for the stomach (*right gastroepiploic artery*) and duodenum (*superior pancreaticoduodenal artery*). The hepatic artery then sends a small *right gastric artery* to the right side of the lesser curvature and continues into the liver.

The right gastroepiploic artery anastomoses with the left gastroepiploic on the greater curvature. This illustrates an arrangement seen also all along the intestines, where most adjacent arteries anastomose, forming a series of arches, or loops.

5. The stomach can be left in place, helping to conserve moisture in the tissues, but it may now be removed if that is desired. For removal a cut should be made across the pyloric limb and another across the last part of the oesophagus and the blood-vessels should be severed close to the stomach. This facilitates examination of the liver, the largest gland of the body, which is an outgrowth of the lining of the alimentary canal and is functionally an important part of the digestive system.

The *liver* has a complex structural pattern but may be regarded as essentially a mass of minute glandular tubules (bile capillaries) all emptying ultimately into a common bile duct and intimately interlaced with innumerable, relatively wide blood-capillaries (sinusoids). The cells composing the bile capillaries pour into these the bile, which is a mixture of various substances, the most important being the bile salts and the bile pigments. The pigments are waste removed from the blood, the salts help to neutralize the acid coming from the stomach, to emulsify fats in the intestinal contents, and to catalyze the action of the pancreatic ferments. The other most conspicuous function of the liver is the storage of carbohydrates brought to it from the alimentary canal. These are removed from the blood and held in the form of glycogen, which can be turned back to the more soluble glucose and restored to the blood as the tissues of the body require it. Fat is also stored, as is an antianaemic substance. Nitrogen-containing waste substances are removed from the blood and made over into the chemical condition (mainly urea) in which they can be returned to the circulation for final excretion by the kidneys. A substance (heparin) which prevents coagulation of the blood is produced in the liver and this organ is one of the minor situations where red blood-cells are destroyed and where the development of new ones takes place.

The liver of the rabbit is divided by a deep median cleft into right and left lobes and each of these is again divided into anterior and posterior lobules. On the right side, the posterior lobule lies close to the dorsal body wall and against the kidney, where it may be hidden by the intestines, and is separated from the anterior lobule by a wide depression in which lies the pyloric limb of the stomach. Caudal to the base of the posterior left lobule is a distinct circular lobe with a thick stalk, the caudate lobe.

A thin-walled sac, the *gall bladder,* lies in a deep depression in the caudal surface of the right anterior lobule. It connects only with the common bile duct, by the *cystic duct.*

All the lobes of the liver are continuous in a common dorsal mass, along the ventral surface of which the very large *portal* vein runs in a deep groove, the *portal fissure.* The portal fissure branches into each of the lobes, containing branches of the portal vein and the *hepatic artery* and tributaries of the *common bile duct.* The common bile duct carries the bile to the superior portion of the duodenum.

The hepatic artery may be traced from the coeliac artery. The portal vein may be seen to be formed by the union of all the veins from the intestines and the stomach and its branching into the various lobules of the liver may be demonstrated by probing. The marked difference in the sizes of the artery and the vein should be noted in relation to the functions of the liver referred to above.

The remnant of the lesser omentum (hepatoduodenal ligament) containing the common bile duct and the vessels to the liver should now be severed and the sheets of peritoneum attaching the anterior surface of the liver to the diaphragm should be divided. A very large vein crosses the dorsal surface of the liver from behind and penetrates the diaphragm. This is the *inferior caval vein,* which should be cut just before and behind the liver so that a piece of it imbedded in a deep groove in the dorsal surface of the liver may now be removed from the body along with that organ. This piece of the inferior caval vein should be opened lengthwise, after which procedure the entrances to it of the *hepatic veins,* the vessels that carry the blood from the liver substance, may be observed.

6. If the duodenal loop described above is spread out without tearing the mesentery, the latter (mesoduodenum) is seen to contain arteries, veins, and a very diffuse mass of brown, glandular material. This glandular material is the main part of the *pancreas,* an extension of which spreads across dorsal to the stomach, where it may have been damaged. The terminal portion of the *duct of the pancreas,* which actually is continuous throughout the organ, may be found leaving it and entering the posterior part of the ascending limb of the duodenum. The duct is thus far removed from the bile duct, which enters the superior portion of the duodenum, in contrast with the condition in many animals (such as man), where the two are close together or even have a common opening.

A small lymph-gland frequently occurs in the more caudal part of the mesoduodenum and in favourable cases lymph-vessels may be observed as delicate, irregular, whitish lines.

All these structures may be more or less imbedded in fat.

7. The intestines may be moved about so as to display the other parts of the mesentery with the contained blood- and lymph-vessels. The large *superior mesenteric artery* will be visible leaving the aorta and branching in a complicated manner to the intestines. Applied to its left side is an extensive mass of lymph-glands.

Other organs which should be noted at this stage, though they are not parts of the digestive system, are the spleen and the collateral ganglia of the sympathetic system.

The *spleen* is an elongate body of considerable size which lies dorsal to the left side of the greater curvature of the stomach and should still be in place after removal of the stomach. It belongs to the vascular system.

Three sympathetic ganglia are to be observed in the mesentery. The more anterior should have been exposed in clearing the origin of the coeliac artery and the superior mesenteric artery as directed in section 4 above. A small, curved, grey-brown body lying against the left side of the superior mesenteric artery is the *superior mesenteric ganglion.* Slightly cephaloventral to it, between the two arteries, is situated another similar body, the *coeliac ganglion,* which is usually somewhat triangular in form. The ganglia are connected and from each run bundles of delicate threads to the neighbouring blood-vessels, which they accompany, mainly to the stomach and intestines. The ganglia receive impulses from the central nervous system through the *greater splanchnic nerve,* a delicate thread emerging from under the diaphragm and crossing the aorta obliquely. (For its origin see page 84.)

Considerably nearer the tail, the *inferior mesenteric artery* will be seen to pass through the mesentery to the descending colon and just in front of this artery, in the dorsal part of the mesentery, appears the very slender, curved, *inferior mesenteric ganglion.* Fibres from this run to the descending colon and to adjacent blood-vessels.

These three ganglia are one of the important factors in nervous regulation of the digestive system.

Just caudolateral to the origin of the superior mesenteric artery, the left *suprarenal gland* lies flattened against the dorsal body wall. It is nearly a quarter of an inch long and much more massive than the ganglia and has a prominent role in regulating the activities of the body by means of chemical substances (hormones) poured into the blood-stream. The best-known of these hormones is adrenalin, produced in the central, or medullary portion of the gland. Adrenalin stimulates activity and prepares the animal in various ways to make sudden effort or to meet emergencies.

8. The intestines may be left in place but if it is desired to remove them the mesentery should now be cut close to the intestines, so as to leave most of its contained structures in place. The descending colon should then be severed near its termination and the intestines should be taken out of the body.

Examination of the anterior and posterior extremities of the digestive system must be delayed until certain other parts are studied.

Chapter XII

URINOGENITAL SYSTEM

As a result of their manner of development, which involves the utilization by the genital system of ducts belonging to or derived from the urinary system, these systems have to be considered together. In the adult mammal, however, only the terminal portions remain common, so that it is convenient to consider first the parts which are concerned only with the removal of liquid, mainly nitrogenous wastes.

A. Urinary Organs

1. The kidneys are the essential excretory organs of this system, the organs which actually extract the waste substances in solution from the blood. Each is a smooth, bean-shaped organ closely pressed against the dorsal body-wall, only its ventral surface being covered by peritoneum. The right kidney lies nearer the head than the left in the rabbit (the opposite of the human situation). An accumulation of fat in the subperitoneal connective tissue frequently forms a rather indefinite *adipose capsule.* Completely surrounding the kidney and directly applied to it is a thin but tough *fibrous coat.* These investments should be removed from one kidney.

The *renal artery* enters a depression, the *renal hilus,* in the medial side of the kidney and the *renal vein* leaves the kidney just caudal to the entrance of the artery.

The *ureter* is a large duct which carries the urine from the kidney to the *urinary bladder.* It leaves the kidney at the hilus and runs directly caudad to enter the dorsal wall of the bladder. The latter lies in the most posterior part of the abdominal cavity and is usually found tightly contracted though it is capable of considerable distension. Along each side of the bladder run an *umbilical artery* and a *vesical vein.*

2. The kidney which has been freed should be divided into dorsal and ventral halves by a horizontal cut beginning where the vessels enter the hilus.

On the cut surface it will be seen that there is a funnel-like internal cavity which narrows into the ureter at the hilus. Into this cavity, the *renal pelvis,* there projects from the more lateral portion

68

of the organ a solid cone of kidney tissue, the *renal papilla*. Invisibly to the naked eye, the surface of the papilla is pierced by the microscopic tubules which pour the excreted liquid into the pelvis.

The outer part of the kidney, the *cortical substance,* is usually distinct in colour and texture from the more central part (including the papilla), which is known as the *medullary substance* and often has a finely striated appearance.

The other kidney may be cut transversly for comparison.

B. Genital Organs—Male

The skin should be cut in the ventral median line from the abdominal cavity back to the tip of the penis and should be stripped away from either side of that organ and to a point lateral to each of the paired *scrotal sacs.* These are sacs containing the testes, the glands which produce the male reproductive elements, or spermatozoa.

If one scrotal sac is opened longitudinally its wall will be seen to be composed of the skin, the subcutaneous connective tissue, a thin layer of muscle (the *cremaster muscle*), and a lining, the *parietal layer of the tunica vaginalis propria.* Each sac has been developed as an evagination of the abdominal cavity and, in the rabbit, retains a connection with it by a narrow canal through which the tunica vaginalis propria is continuous with the peritoneum. Like the peritoneum, the tunica vaginalis is an uninterrupted sheet, the testis being covered by it so as, strictly speaking, to remain outside the cavity. The portion of the tunica vaginalis on the surface of the testis is the *visceral layer* and this is continuous with the parietal layer through a double sheet, the *mesorchium,* which is directly comparable with mesentery.

At its cephalic end the elongate, elliptical *testis* is invested by the cap-like *head of the epididymis,* which is usually more or less covered by the base of a small conical mass of fat. The head is composed of coiled microscopic tubules and forms the beginning of the epididymis, the first portion of the passage carrying spermatozoa from the testis. It is continued as a slender band, the *body of the epididymis,* along the side of the testis and expands at the caudal end into a thicker mass, the *tail of the epididymis.* The last is intimately bound to the side of a short cord of connective tissue, the *gubernaculum,* by which the testis is attached to the end of the scrotal sac.

Doubling back on its course, the duct constituting the tail of the epididymis continues without interruption as the *ductus de-*

ferens, which passes along beside the mesorchium, runs through the passage into the abdominal cavity and curves across the ureter to enter the ventral wall of the base of a small sac, the *seminal vesicle,* dorsal to the urinary bladder.

The principal blood-supply of the testis is by the *internal spermatic artery,* which rises from the aorta and enters the scrotum through the passage from the abdominal cavity. Beside it runs the spermatic vein.

C. Organs both Urinary and Genital—Male

1. Clearing away the skin and connective tissue round the *penis* reveals it as a whitish, hard, rod-like structure with a softer band running along its dorsal side to a terminal opening. The softer band is the *urethra,* a tubular passage for liquid, which contains in its ventral wall the harder, paired *cavernous bodies.* The latter are elongate masses of spongy tissue connected with the blood-vessels (erectile tissue) and surrounded by very thick, tough, fibrous sheaths which give the hardness to the organ. The paired character of the cavernous bodies is not evident externally but *after the study of the system has been completed* the penis should be cut transversely, when the relations of the two bodies and the urethra will be readily visible on the cut surface (Fig. 20).

At their proximal ends the two cavernous bodies diverge to be attached to the posteroventral edges of the respective ischia. The divergent ends constitute the *crura penis.* A single, thinner, median cord, the *suspensory ligament,* attaches the ventral surface of the penis to the caudal end of the pelvic symphysis.

Each of these ligaments is partly concealed by a muscle. Ventral to the suspensory ligament, and attached through it, lies the *pubocavernosus muscle* and superficial to each crus is an *ischiocavernosus muscle.*

The foregoing muscles and ligaments must now be severed at their attachments to the pelvic girdle and the pelvic symphysis must be divided by a median, longitudinal incision. The two halves of the pelvic girdle are then to be spread apart and everything holding the urinogenital organs and the rectum in place is to be severed. These organs in their entirety can then be removed from the body as a single piece. Afterwards the rectum should be separated from the remaining parts.

2. It is now possible to see the continuous passage, the *urethra,* from the urinary bladder to the external opening at the tip of the

penis. The first or *prostatic portion* of this is characterized by its association with the genital ducts. It receives the opening of the seminal vesicle, a flat glandular sac lying just dorsal to the base of the bladder. Into the thin ventral wall of this sac, close to its connection with the urethra, open the deferent ducts. The dorsal wall of the seminal vesicle is largely occupied by the rather massive, whitish *prostate gland.* Immediately caudal to the prostate a pair of *bulbourethral glands* forms a bilobed swelling in the dorsal wall of the urethra. All these glands and two others (vesicular and para- prostate) contribute to the liquid vehicle for the spermatozoa. (The seminal vesicle is probably not a reservoir for storing spermatozoa, as is often stated.)

After the short prostatic portion the urethra continues as the longer, thin-walled, *membranous portion* and then traverses the penis as the *cavernous portion.*

D. Genital Organs—Female

In contrast with the testes of the male, which, during develop- ment, have been displaced caudally into saccular evaginations from the abdominal cavity, the essential reproductive glands of the

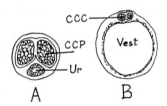

Fig. 20. Diagrams of transverse sections of the penis (A) and the vestibulum (B). ccc, cavernous body of the clitoris; ccp, cavernous body of the penis; Ur, male urethra; Vest, vestibulum of female.

female, the *ovaries,* have migrated very little from their original position on the dorsal wall of the abdomen. There they appear as a pair of small, elongated, elliptical bodies. Often they are marked by translucent or dark spots, vesicular ovarian follicles.

Each ovary is covered by peritoneum and connected to the body- wall by a peritoneal fold, the *mesovarium,* through which it receives the *internal spermatic artery.*

Just lateral to each ovary lies a narrow *uterine tube,* which bends round in a hook-like fashion from its beginning in a broad, thin- walled funnel. This funnel, usually collapsed in the embalmed animal, is open to the abdominal cavity but more or less envelops the ovary so that an ovum discharged into the cavity is almost sure to enter the funnel. Caudally the uterine tube expands suddenly into the much wider and longer *uterus,* the size of which varies enormously according to the reproductive history of the individual.

The uterine tube and the uterus are supported by a peritoneal fold known as the *broad ligament,* which is continuous with the mesovarium. Across this runs a secondary fold, the *ovarian ligament,* from the ovary to the beginning of the uterus, whence it continues as the *round ligament* to a pit (the *vaginal sac*) near the caudal end of the ventral abdominal wall. This fold and pit correspond respectively to the gubernaculum and the scrotal sac of the male.

The two uteri open separately into the anterior end of a single, wide, muscular, median tube, the *vagina.*

E. Organs both Urinary and Genital—Female

1. The median ventral incision of the skin should be extended back from the abdominal cavity to the external urinogenital opening and the skin and connective tissue should be cleared away so as to reveal a small, flexible, white rod in a median position. This rod is the *clitoris.* It lies in the ventral wall of a wide, soft tube, the *vestibulum,* which is a passage for both urinary and reproductive materials, corresponding with the distal part of the urethra in the male. The clitoris is composed of paired *cavernous bodies,* homologous with those of the penis and made up, like them, of erectile tissue surrounded by a thick, fibrous sheath so tough as to make the clitoris feel hard. The paired character of the cavernous bodies may be revealed *after the study of the system has been completed* by cutting across the organ and examining the cut surfaces (Fig. 20).

The proximal ends of the two cavernous bodies diverge as the *crura clitoridis* and are attached to the posterior edge of the pelvic girdle. The crura are largely concealed by a pair of muscles superficial to them, the *ischiocavernosus muscles.* A single, thinner, median cord, the *suspensory ligament,* attaches the body of the clitoris to the caudal end of the pelvic symphysis, and ventral to this lies a small, spindle-shaped, *pubocavernosus muscle.* All these parts correspond with those of the male.

The muscles and ligaments just described are now to be severed at their attachments to the ischia and the pelvic girdle is to be divided by a median, longitudinal cut through the thin plate of cartilage forming the pelvic symphysis. If the halves of the girdle are then pressed apart, the connective tissue and any other parts holding the rectum and the urinogenital organs in place being severed, these organs may now be removed from the body in a single piece. The rectum should then be separated from the urino-genital ducts.

2. The passage from the bladder and the vagina to the exterior may now be examined. Within the pelvic cavity, the vagina is joined ventrally by a short passage, the *urethra,* leading from the urinary bladder. A wide duct, the *vestibulum,* common to the urinary and reproductive systems, then leads straight to the external opening. The vestibulum has the clitoris imbedded in the ventral wall of its terminal portion. It is relatively much longer in the rabbit than in some animals.

The urethra and the vestibulum of the female together correspond with the passage known as urethra in the male. On the dorsal wall of the vestibulum is situated a *bulbourethral gland* which helps to lubricate the interior of the passage but the other glands present in this region of the male do not occur in the female.

The vestibulum and the vagina may be opened by a longitudinal incision, which will reveal the opening of the urethra into the vestibulum and the openings of the two uteri into the vagina.

Chapter XIII

WALLS OF THE THORAX AND MECHANISM OF BREATHING

A. Diaphragm

The abdominal cavity is separated from the thoracic cavity in front of it by a transverse muscular partition, the diaphragm, which is one of the distinctive features of mammals. The partition has a markedly curved form so that in a quadrupedal mammal it is like a bowl set on edge, with its concavity facing backward and accommodating the smooth, rounded, anterior surface of the liver and its convexity bulging into the cavity of the thorax.

Structurally the diaphragm consists of a broad ring of radially-arranged muscle surrounding a central tendinous area. The muscle has origin on the internal surface of the sternum (*sternal portion of the diaphragm*), on the internal surfaces of the seven posterior ribs (*costal portion*), and on median, ventral processes of the first three lumbar vertebrae (*lumbar portion*).

The lumbar portion is composed of two thickened and elongate muscular bands, the *crura,* of which the right is much larger than the left and between which the aorta emerges through the *hiatus aorticus.*

All three portions of the muscle have their insertion in the *tendinous centre,* which is pulled caudad by their contraction so that the abdominal viscera are pushed back and the thoracic cavity is enlarged.

The tendinous centre is pierced by the oesophagus and by the inferior vena cava, which is somewhat asymmetrically placed, the vein being a little to the right and ventral to the oesophagus.

B. Ventral and Lateral Walls

The ventral and lateral walls should be cleared by removal of the pectoral muscles and the anterior limbs on both sides, the *ribs* and the *external intercostal muscles* being thereby exposed.

The external intercostal muscles have their origins on the posterior margins of the bone-ribs and their insertions on the anterior edges of the succeeding bone-ribs. They thus leave unoccupied the spaces between the costal cartilages, where the *internal intercostal muscles* are consequently visible, since the latter muscles extend from both bony and cartilaginous parts of each rib to those of the next.

The oblique orientation of the ribs should be noted, this being such that contraction of the intercostal muscles pulls them into a more nearly transverse position and thereby increases both the dorsoventral diameter and the transverse diameter of the thoracic

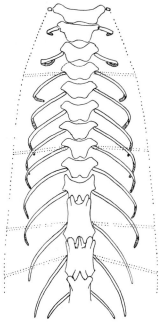

FIG. 21. Diagram of a dorsal view of the thoracic skeleton to show the position of the ribs at rest (or in expiration) and in inspiration.

cavity. Occurring simultaneously with the contraction of the diaphragm, which increases the length of the cavity, these movements tend to produce a potential vacuum and so draw air into the lungs.

Thus the diaphragmatic and intercostal muscles are the main agents for inspiration, or the intake of air in breathing. Expiration is accomplished largely by the elastic reaction of the tissues when these muscles relax, assisted by the contraction of the abdominal muscles, of small *transverse thoracic muscles* which originate on the sternum and are inserted on the ventral parts of the ribs, and of minute involuntary muscles in the walls of the smaller airpassages.

An incision may now be made on the right side from the middle of the first bone-rib to the ventral end of the ninth. A more dorsal longitudinal incision on the left side and a transverse cut connecting these just in front of the diaphragm permits removal of the ventral and left lateral walls, in which the internal intercostal and the transverse thoracic muscles mentioned above may be observed.

Examination of the essential respiratory organs and the air-passages is best postponed until some of the other contents of the thorax have been studied.

Chapter XIV

HEART AND PRINCIPAL BLOOD-VESSELS

1. *Thymus gland*

In the anteroventral part of the thorax appears an irregularly triangular brownish mass of fatty consistency, the thymus gland. This is an endocrine gland which is important during growth and development, though its precise functions are still obscure. It is gradually reduced about the time of maturity but usually retains considerable size in the rabbit (Fig. 23).

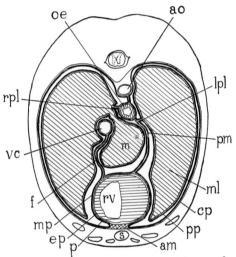

Fig. 22. Diagram of a transverse section of the thorax of a rabbit, passing through the posterior tip of the heart. From *Bensley's Practical Anatomy of the Rabbit.* am, anterior mediastinum; ao, aorta; cp, costal pleura; ep epicardium; f, fold of mediastinal pleura containing the inferior caval vein; lpl, left pulmonary ligament; m, medial lobule of inferior lobe of right lung; ml, middle lobe of the left lung; mp, mediastinal pleura; oe, oesophagus; p, pericardium; pm, posterior mediastinum; pp, pulmonary pleura; rpl, right pulmonary ligament; rv, right ventricle; s, sternum; vc, inferior caval vein.

The thymus should be carefully removed without injury to underlying structures.

2. *Pericardium*

The heart may be seen partly dorsal and caudal to the thymus.

77

surrounded by a loose, membranous sac. The cavity of the sac, the *pericardial cavity,* is one of four derived from the original body cavity, or coelom, the others being the two pleural cavities, which contain the lungs, and the abdominal cavity. The pericardial cavity is enclosed by an unbroken sheet of smooth, moist epithelium supported by connective tissue, which is closely applied to the surface of the heart as the *visceral layer* and lines the outer wall of the sac as the *parietal layer,* these being continuous at the attached base of the heart. Cutting open the pericardial sac reveals the heart itself with the visceral layer of the pericardium forming its outer surface.

3. *External features of the heart*

The larger part of the heart is the tapering, caudal, *ventricular portion,* comprising the very massive, muscular, *left ventricle* and the visibly thinner-walled *right ventricle.*

Craniolaterally appear the still much thinner-walled *left atrium* and *right atrium.* (The thinness of their walls may be obscured by their being filled with firm masses of coagulated blood.)

The right ventricle appears to be continued forward between the atria, ventrally, as the *pulmonary artery.* This vessel turns dorsad

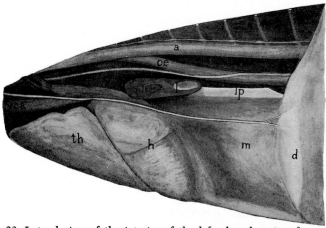

Fig. 23. Lateral view of the interior of the left pleural cavity after removal of the left thoracic wall and the lung. From *Bensley's Practical Anatomy of the Rabbit.* a, thoracic aorta; d, diaphragm; h, heart enclosed by pericardium; l, remnant of hilus of left lung; lp, pulmonary ligament; m, posterior mediastinum (partition between right and left pleural cavities); oe, oesophagus; th, thymus gland; vca, left superior caval vein; The phrenic nerve is visible crossing the pericardium and the mediastinum and branching into the diaphragm. More dorsally the vagus nerve crosses the lateral surface of the oesophagus and the sympathetic trunk appears on the dorsal wall.

and then caudad and bifurcates dorsal to the heart into right and left pulmonary arteries.

The left ventricle is similarly continued forward into the *aorta,* which passes dorsal to the pulmonary artery and then, as the *arch of the aorta,* curves round towards the left and dorsad.

The muscular wall of the heart is supplied by a pair of small *coronary arteries* and drained by cardiac veins, of which the arteries at least should be visible on the surface.

The blood which is to be pumped out through the pulmonary artery is brought to the heart through several large veins. The inferior vena cava (or inferior caval vein) comes from behind and, passing dorsal to the ventricle enters the caudal end of the right atrium. The left superior vena cava comes from the left side of the neck and crosses the dorsal surface of the heart to empty into the right atrium near the entrance of the inferior caval vein. The right superior caval vein passes directly into the anterior end of the right atrium. These carry deoxygenated blood from all parts of the body.

Aerated blood is conveyed from the lungs by pulmonary veins which usually unite into two main vessels from each side, all four entering the left atrium caudodorsally.

4. *Internal features of the heart*

The heart may be removed by dividing the large veins and arteries just described, the aorta being severed just before it gives off its first large branch (the innominate artery). Care must be taken to avoid damaging other structures dorsal to the heart.

The right ventricle should be opened by a longitudinal incision of the ventral wall, the incision being carried forward along the pulmonary artery.

The inner surface of the ventricular wall has prominent muscular ridges, the *trabeculae carneae.*

The *right atrioventricular (tricuspid) valve* appears mainly as a thin, membranous flap projecting backwards from the ventral edge of the atrioventricular opening. In the rabbit there is also a much reduced dorsal flap but a third flap, to justify the name tricuspid, is absent.

From the free edge of the flap delicate but strong threads (*chordae tendineae*) extend to the tips of prominent projections from the muscular wall opposite, the *papillary muscles.* When the ventricle contracts, the pressure of blood sweeps the flap across the atrioventricular opening but the chordae tendineae prevent its being carried right through, so that the passage is effectively stopped. The papillary muscles exert appropriate tension so that this will be true at all stages of contraction of the ventricle. On the other hand, when the ventricle relaxes, pressure of the blood from the atrium pushes the flap aside passively and allows unobstructed flow.

Another set of valves, the *semilunar valves,* is situated at the entrance to the pulmonary artery. These also work passively, being three simple, membranous pockets opening towards the artery so that they offer no obstacle to blood entering it. Any tendency to back-flow, however, at once fills the pockets so that their edges meet and close the aperture.

If the left ventricle is similarly opened, corresponding *left atrioventricular (bicuspid* or *mitral) valves* and *aortic semilunar valves* will be observed.

In specimens injected with latex a very perfect cast of the arch of the aorta and the cavities of the semilunar valves is often formed. This may be drawn out of the vessel after removal of the heart from the body and the origins of the coronary arteries in two of the three valvular cavities may then be seen conveniently.

5. *Aorta and its primary branches*

(a) The *arch of the aorta* begins at the anterior end of the heart, where it represents part of the ventral aorta of embryos and of lower vertebrates, and then curves to the left and dorsad to turn back along the internal surfaces of the left ribs and reach the median plane, ventral to the thoracic vertebrae. A short, thick cord, the *arterial ligament,* attaches it to the beginning of the left pulmonary artery. This is a remnant of a foetal connection, the ductus arteriosus, which is derived from the most posterior branchial arterial arch of the embryo. The aortic arch is crossed ventrally by the left superior vena cava, which should not be destroyed in exposing the aorta. The portion of the dorsal aorta contained within the thorax is called the thoracic aorta, its continuation caudad in the abdominal cavity being the abdominal aorta.

(b) After the small coronary arteries, noted above, the first branch of the aorta is the *innominate artery,* a short vessel which divides into the *right subclavian* and *right common carotid arteries* to the right anterior limb and the right side of the neck and head respectively. The *left common carotid artery* originates from the convex anterior surface of the aortic arch just beyond the innominate or may rise from the latter. The *left subclavian artery* leaves the arch further along. Each subclavian artery gives off a group of important branches to the neck and thorax before passing into the axillary fossa, where it is given the name *axillary artery*.

(*c*) By gently raising the left lung, the dissector may follow the aorta caudad through the thorax, in which it gives off a regular series of paired *intercostal arteries* between the ribs from the fourth intercostal space back. (The first three intercostal arteries rise from a single branch of the subclavian at each side.)

(*d*) After the aorta passes through the diaphragm, its abdominal portion gives off branches which are classified as a *parietal series* to the body wall and a *visceral series* to the internal organs.

The parietal series includes very small *superior phrenic arteries* to the diaphragm, rising in the hiatus aorticus by a common trunk; seven pairs of *lumbar arteries*, each pair rising by a common trunk from the dorsal wall of the aorta opposite one of the lumbar vertebrae; and the *median sacral artery*, really the direct continuation of the aorta itself, which rises from the dorsal wall of the latter and continues it along the sacral and caudal regions. The seventh pair of lumbar arteries rises from the median sacral instead of from the aorta itself. *Suprarenolumbar arteries* to the wall cephalolateral to the kidneys rise not from the aorta but from the renal arteries.

The visceral series of branches of the abdominal aorta comprises the unpaired, ventral, *coeliac, superior mesenteric,* and *inferior mesenteric arteries* to the digestive organs and the paired, lateral, *renal arteries* to the kidneys and *internal spermatic arteries* to the gonads.

The abdominal aorta ends at the level of the seventh lumbar vertebra by bifurcating into the large *common iliac arteries*.

(*e*) Each common iliac artery is a short trunk which soon divides into a large *external iliac artery* continuing directly into the limb, where it is known as the femoral artery, and a smaller, backward-directed *hypogastric artery* (internal iliac) which supplies branches to the walls and contents of the pelvic region. The umbilical artery, observed on the urinary bladder, originates from the beginning of the hypogastric artery. The *sciatic artery* is a continuation of the hypogastric.

The first branch of the common iliac artery is usually the *iliolumbar* artery to the body wall but this often appears as one of the parietal branches of the aorta itself.

6. *The systemic veins*

The right and left superior caval veins may be followed forward into the base of the neck, where each is formed by the junction of a large *external jugular,* a slightly smaller *subclavian* (from the anterior limb), and a much smaller, deep *internal jugular vein,* the jugulars carrying all the blood from the head and neck.

A little in front of this junction the external jugular veins of the two sides are connected by a *transverse jugular vein,* which is significant because in many mammals it becomes the sole passage for blood from the left jugular and subclavian veins, the left superior caval vein disappearing.

The inferior vena cava may be traced back from its ending in the right atrium through the right pleural cavity, where it lies in a fold projecting from the median partition separating the two pleural cavities and is accommodated in a deep groove in the ventral surface of the right lung (Fig. 22). It receives no tributaries in the thorax but as it passes through the diaphragm it is joined by a pair of *inferior phrenic veins* from that muscle.

Behind the diaphragm the inferior vena cava has been interrupted by the removal of the liver, in the dorsal part of which it was imbedded and from which it received the hepatic veins. It may be followed caudad close to the right side of the abdominal aorta, receiving *renal veins, lumbar veins, spermatic veins,* and *iliolumbar veins* corresponding with the similarly-named arteries. (In the male the left spermatic vein normally runs forward to join the vena cava at the termination of the renal vein.)

The inferior caval vein is considered to commence dorsal to the posterior end of the aorta where the two *external iliac veins* from the limbs join the *common hypogastric,* a short median vessel formed by union of the *paired hypogastric veins* from the sacral region.

Chapter XV

PERIPHERAL NERVES IN THE TRUNK

A. Somatic Nerves

The central nervous system is connected with the trunk and limbs by a segmental series of spinal nerves each containing large numbers of both afferent and efferent nerve fibres. (The terms afferent and efferent are to be preferred to sensory and motor because all afferent impulses do not produce conscious sensation and all efferent impulses do not produce movement.) Each nerve emerges from the vertebral column between two vertebrae and breaks into certain primary branches of which the largest is a *ventral branch.* The ventral branches of the last five cervical and the first thoracic spinal nerves form a network, the *brachial plexus,* through which the anterior limb is innervated and which has been described in the chapter on that limb.

1. If the inner surface of the thoracic wall is now examined, the remaining ventral branches of the thoracic nerves, the *intercostal nerves,* may be observed beside the arteries on the intercostal muscles.

Also belonging to the somatic group but rising in the neck, chiefly from the fourth cervical nerves, the *phrenic nerves* traverse the thorax longitudinally along the sides of the pericardium. The left nerve continues along the median septum behind the pericardium to end in the diaphragm (Fig. 23). The right phrenic nerve lies parallel to the inferior caval vein in the thorax and ends similarly.

2. The regular series of spinal nerves may be followed back in the abdomen, where the *lumbar nerves* are visible crossing the dorsal wall obliquely. The last four lumbar nerves, the sacral nerves, and the first caudal nerve are connected near their proximal ends to form a network, the *lumbosacral plexus,* which supplies the nerves to the posterior limb just as the brachial plexus does to the anterior limb. As a rule the femoral nerve is formed mainly from the fifth, sixth, and seventh lumbar nerves, the sciatic from the last lumbar and first sacral nerves.

83

B. Visceral Nerves

The peripheral nervous structures controlling the activities of the visceral organs are known as the autonomic system and this is considered to comprise sympathetic and parasympathetic subdivisions. Most visceral organs receive nerve-fibres from both of these, their effects being sometimes supplementary but frequently antagonistic. The connections of the sympathetic system with the central nervous organs are through the thoracic and lumbar spinal nerves, those of the parasympathetic system through certain cranial and sacral nerves.

These autonomic pathways differ from the somatic peripheral pathways in that each nerve-fibre leaving the central nervous organs is interrupted at some point on its way to the periphery and there passes the impulses to a new nerve cell. Such cells usually have their bodies grouped into little masses, or *ganglia,* so that the autonomic system differs grossly from the somatic nerves in having ganglia at various points (Fig. 25, p. 98).

The sympathetic portion of the autonomic system may advantageously be examined at this stage of the dissection.

1. If the left lung is carefully raised and the dorsal wall of the thorax examined, the *thoracic portion of the left sympathetic trunk* may be observed as a very delicate thread running along the lateral surfaces of the bodies of the vertebrae. A minute, spindle-shaped ganglion lies against or slightly cephalic to the base of each rib (Fig. 23). An exceedingly fine *ramus communicans* connects each ganglion with the corresponding spinal nerve and threads too delicate to be readily dissected pass from the ganglia to the organs in the thoracic cavity, running along the blood-vessels.

The *splanchnic nerve* rises in the more posterior thoracic ganglia, usually starting about the eighth, and runs along the dorsal wall and through the diaphragm to end mainly in the coeliac and superior mesenteric ganglia (p. 66), which regulate the stomach and most of the intestine through nerves-plexuses following the coeliac and superior mesenteric arteries.

2. The sympathetic trunk continues into the abdominal region, where it lies dorsal to the aorta, close to the common trunks of the lumbar arteries, the ganglia being slightly anterior or lateral to these. Again rami communicantes connect the ganglia with the spinal nerves. The lumbar portion of the trunk includes seven ganglia, the sacral portion four, and a very delicate caudal portion has two ganglia and ends in a median ganglion in which terminates

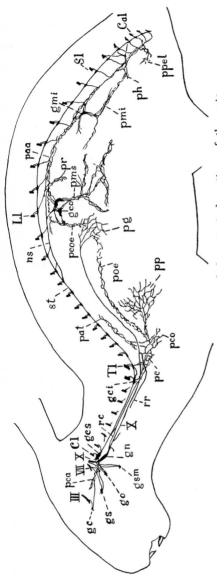

Fig. 24. Diagrammatic lateral view of the principal portions of the autonomic nervous system, from *Bensley's Practical Anatomy of the Rabbit*. In the case of paired structures only those of the left side are shown. Cl, first cervical nerve; Cal, first caudal nerve; Ll, first lumbar nerve; Sl, first sacral nerve; Tl, first thoracic nerve; III, oculomotor nerve; VII, facial nerve; X, vagus nerve; gc, ciliary ganglion; gci, inferior cervical sympathetic ganglion; gco, coeliac ganglion; gcs, superior cervical sympathetic ganglion; gmi, inferior mesenteric ganglion; gn, ganglion nodosum; go, otic ganglion; gs, sphenopalatine ganglion; gsm, submaxillary ganglion; ns, greater splanchnic nerve; paa, abdominal aortic plexus; pat, thoracic aortic plexus; pc, cardiac plexus; pca, carotid plexus; pco, coronary plexus; pcoe, coeliac plexus; pg, gastric plexus; ph, hypogastric plexus; pmi, inferior mesenteric plexus; pms, superior mesenteric plexus; poe, oesophageal plexus; pp, pulmonary plexus; ppel, plexuses in pelvic viscera; pr, renal plexus; rc, cardiac branch of the vagus nerve; rr, recurrent branch of the vagus nerve; st, sympathetic trunk.

also the trunk of the other side. Nerves from these ganglia, too delicate to be seen in gross dissection, are distributed to the visceral organs in the form of plexuses surrounding the blood-vessels. An unpaired, slender, elongate, *inferior mesenteric ganglion* in the mesentery in front of the inferior mesenteric artery is also involved in this.

3. Anteriorly the thoracic portion of the left sympathetic trunk passes dorsal to the aortic arch and the first thoracic ganglion, on both right and left sides, is situated just behind the subclavian artery. The trunk then divides, forming a loop, the *ansa subclavia,* round the artery, connecting the first thoracic ganglion with the *inferior cervical ganglion* in front. From here the sympathetic trunk may be traced forward in the neck, just dorsal to the common carotid artery. This artery, already observed leaving the arch of the aorta, should be followed up to the head, to which mainly its branches are distributed. Lateral to the artery lies the vagus nerve and dorsal to the artery, medial to the vagus, is the more slender sympathetic trunk. Medial to this again lies another delicate nerve, the cardiac branch of the vagus. At the base of the head the sympathetic trunk ends in a marked swelling, the *superior cervical ganglion* (the only ganglion in front of the inferior cervical).

4. The *vagus nerve,* noticed incidentally in exposing the sympathetic trunk, belongs to the parasympathetic division of the autonomic system. It is the tenth cranial nerve, connecting with the hindbrain and containing both afferent and efferent fibres. At the cephalic end of the neck the vagus gives off a *superior laryngeal nerve* to the larynx and a *cardiac branch* which courses backward dorsal to the common carotid artery, as noted above. The cardiac branch (also known as the depressor nerve) is an afferent nerve from the heart and aortic arch and can be traced back into a diffuse cardiac plexus in the connective tissue at the base of these organs.

The main left vagus nerve runs caudad dorsal to the superior vena cava and ventral to the arch of the aorta and gives off a *recurrent branch* which turns cephalad dorsal to the arterial ligament and the arch to reach the trachea and the larynx. Near its beginning the recurrent branch sends efferent (inhibitory) fibres for the heart into the cardiac plexus.

The vagus nerve may be followed back dorsal to the pulmonary vessels and the bronchus, where it gives fibres to the lungs, and along the oesophagus to the stomach. It carries excitatory impulses to the stomach, antagonistic to inhibitory impulses reaching that organ from the sympathetic ganglia.

On the right side the relations of the vagus are similar to those on the left except that the recurrent nerve curves round the subclavian artery.

Chapter XVI

RESPIRATORY ORGANS

1. The *lungs* are the essential organs of external respiration, that is the place where oxygen and carbon dioxide are exchanged between the air and the blood, or, to be more precise, the *alveoli*, microscopic sacs within the lungs, are the site of this process.

Each lung is enclosed in a pleural sac comparable with the pericardial and peritoneal sacs, the two pleural sacs being separated by a median partition which contains the oesophagus dorsally and into the cranioventral part of which the pericardium is, as it were, wedged. The lining of each sac is the *pleura*. A roughly transverse fold of pleura, the *pulmonary ligament*, connects the medial edge of each lung to the partition and a more ventral fold on the right side contains the inferior vena cava (Figs. 22 and 23).

If any obscuring parts are still in place, they should now be removed so that the lungs may be observed clearly. The right wall of the thorax may be removed if so desired.

Each lung is a spongy, distensible organ divided by deep fissures into lobes. The right lung is larger and more lobulated than the left. The pulmonary artery and veins and the air-ducts, or *bronchi*, penetrate the medial portion of the lung, known as the *hilus*. The courses of some of the veins are superficial for a short distance but the arteries and bronchi at once penetrate deeply. On the right side, however, the bronchus first divides round the entering artery, sending an *eparterial bronchus* into the superior lobe (the most cephalic) of the lung.

2. Accessory organs of respiration are the breathing mechanism, which has already been described, and the passages through which air flows between the alveoli and the environment.

The bronchial branches and the bronchi themselves are supported by rings of soft, flexible cartilage and the primary bronchi to the two lungs are formed by bifurcation at the cephalic end of the thorax of a median windpipe, the *trachea*, which also is supported by cartilaginous rings. Each tracheal ring, however, is incomplete dorsally, where the trachea fits against the oesophagus.

3. The trachea is largely concealed by the muscles of the neck, which should be examined and then removed.

The *sternomastoid muscles* originate together on the manubrium sterni and are inserted on the mastoid processes of the skull at either side. Singly they turn the head and depress the snout. The slender *sternohyoid muscles* also have a common origin on the cephalic part of the sternum and are in contact along the mid-ventral line of the neck. They are inserted on the greater cornua of the hyoid. Separation and division of the sternohyoids reveals the sternothyreoid muscles, which originate in common with them and are inserted on the thyreoid cartilage of the larynx. The *thyreohyoid muscles* continue from the areas of insertion of the sternothyreoids to the hyoid bone.

4. In the upper part of the neck the trachea is replaced by the "voice-box", or *larynx*. The most conspicuous part of this is the saddle-shaped *thyreoid cartilage*, behind which the *cricoid cartilage* appears like an enlarged and thickened tracheal ring, a small sheet of muscle connecting them.

The larynx and the oesophagus both connect with the pharynx, which is thus common to the respiratory and the digestive systems. Air may pass between the pharynx and the exterior through the nasal passages and through the mouth. Since these do not belong only to the respiratory system and since they require some special dissection, their consideration will be reserved for a later chapter.

5. A rather large, elongate, *deep cervical lymph gland* lies dorso-lateral to the thyreoid cartilage. The *thyreoid gland* is a flattened mass closely applied to the ventral and lateral surfaces of the trachea. Though single in origin, it appears as paired lobes connected by a median isthmus.

The common carotid artery (p. 86) of each side passes cephalad lateral to the trachea, carrying blood to the head. In the neck it gives a *superior thyreoid artery* to the thyreoid gland and adjacent parts and a *laryngeal artery* to the interior of the larynx, etc. The internal jugular vein (p. 82) is situated lateral to the common carotid artery.

The vagus nerve (pp. 86, 104), lateral to the common carotid artery, its cardiac branch, and the sympathetic trunk, both dorsal to the artery, have been noted on page 86. A fourth delicate nerve, the descending branch of the hypoglossal, runs ventral to the artery and supplies the sternohyoid and related muscles.

Chapter XVII

MUSCLES OF MASTICATION

IF the head is to be dissected, it is necessary to examine some of its more superficial structures first. The median ventral incision of the skin should be continued forward to the lower lip and the skin should be stripped away from the head and the neck on one side right round to the mid-dorsal line. The external ear may be severed at its base and the lining of the eyelids cut.

1. The platysma, an exceedingly thin sheet of muscle, covers the ventral and lateral aspects of the head and neck just under the skin and varies in distinctness at different points. There is also an extensive system of thin facial and auricular muscles. The platysma and associated fascia should be cleared away.

2. Two large salivary glands should now be visible

The *parotid gland* is a rather large, finely lobulated, irregular, brownish body closely applied to the posterior margin of the mandible and extending up to the base of the ear. Its duct enters the mouth through the lining of the cheek just anterior to the masseter muscle (3 below).

The *submandibular* ("*submaxillary*") *gland* is smaller, smoothly rounded, often darker, and is situated just ventromedial to the angle of the mandible. Its duct (which pierces the floor of the mouth some distance away) may be seen running dorsad from it.

3. The *masseter muscle* covers the lateral surface of the angle and of the ramus of the mandible, upon which it is inserted. The origin is on the zygomatic arch, partly by a broad, superficial sheet of tendon, and the fibres mostly slant downward and backward. An anterior fleshy portion curves across the ventral margin of the mandible and extends backward as a distinct band along the ventro-medial edge.

A sharp scalpel should be passed along the dorsal margin and the medial surface of the zygomatic arch so as to free it from all attached soft parts except the masseter muscle. The zygomatic processes of both maxilla and squamosal bone being divided, the arch and the whole masseter muscle should then be removed, the latter being cleanly cut from its insertion.

4. The *temporal muscle* is relatively small in the rabbit, being much larger in many other mammals. Its origin is in the temporal fossa of the skull, where it extends over the side of the cranium to near the suture between parietal and occipital bones. The long tendon of insertion passes over the zygomatic process of the squamosal bone, where it is held in place by a ligament, and is inserted on the coronoid process of the mandible.

It is evident that the general action of the masseter muscle is to pull the lower jaw upward and forward, that of the much weaker temporal muscle is to pull it upward and backward.

5. The *digastric muscle* appears as a spindle-shaped mass lying against the anteroventral part of the medial surface of the mandible, being inserted just caudal and caudodorsal to the mandibular symphysis. The muscle (which, despite its name, has only one belly in the rabbit) tapers backwards into a long tendon by which it originates from the jugular process of the occipital bone.

The action of this muscle is to pull the mandible backwards or, with appropriate cooperation from other muscles, to lower it.

6. The *internal pterygoid muscle* covers most of the medial aspect of the mandible caudal to the insertion of the digastric, being inserted on the ventral part of the medial surface of the angle. The origin, on the pterygoid process of the skull, can be observed more readily after displacement of one half of the mandible according to the following procedure. The muscle raises the mandible.

The two halves of the mandible should be separated at the symphysis and the attachment of the lips and the lining of the mouth to the half to be removed should be severed. The insertions of the digastric and internal pterygoid muscles should be divided by cutting along the surface of the ventral part of the bone. In this procedure the *mylohyoid muscle,* a thin transverse sheet which attaches the base of the tongue to the mandible, should also be cut but the incision should not damage the external pterygoid, which is inserted dorsal to the internal pterygoid.

If the zygomatic arch was adequately removed previously, the ventral edge of the mandible can now be rotated laterad and dorsad.

7. The *external pterygoid muscle* comprises two distinct parts. The *superior head* has its origin on the alisphenoid bone behind the pterygoid process and its insertion on the medial surface of the ramus of the mandible, where its area is marked by a distinct depression. The *inferior head* is practically at right angles to the foregoing, having origin on the pterygoid process and insertion on the anterior and medial aspects of the neck of the mandible.

The superior head mainly raises the mandible while the inferior head pulls it forward, the differentiation of the latter being related to the back-and-forth movement in chewing and gnawing.

8. The *inferior alveolar artery,* the *inferior alveolar vein,* and the *inferior alveolar nerve,* which are related to the lower teeth, pass through the mandibular foramen and run between the external and internal pterygoid muscles.

CHAPTER XVIII

ORAL CAVITY, PHARYNX, AND LARYNX

THE displaced half of the mandible may now be removed entirely and the two pterygoid muscles may be separated from their origins and also removed. A probe should be inserted into the mouth and pushed back into the oesophagus, care being taken not to pass it into the larynx. An incision should then be made, following the probe, through the lateral walls of the oral cavity, the pharynx, and the beginning of the oesophagus. The ventral organs may be pulled down so as to open the cavities better.

1. The *oral cavity* is considered to include the *vestibulum oris,* between the lips and cheeks and the teeth and jaws, and the *oral cavity proper* internal to the jaws.

2. The *pharynx* continues the passage backward from the oral cavity without any definite boundary between them being recognizable in the adult. It may transmit both food and air from the oral cavity and also receives air from the nasal fossae.

3. The roof of the oral cavity is formed anteriorly by the bony *hard palate,* which is covered by a tough mucous membrane with prominent transverse ridges. It is continued caudad by the *soft palate,* a thin, fleshy membrane without bony support which extends back through the pharynx.

The soft palate divides the pharynx into a dorsal *nasopharynx* and a ventral *oropharynx,* which unite behind the palate in a short *laryngeal portion,* this in turn leading to the oesophagus and the larynx.

4. The tongue is a massive, muscular organ attached basally to the hyoid bone and projecting over the whole floor of the mouth. It is attached to the floor anteriorly by a median fold, the *frenulum linguae.* The tongue is covered dorsally by very fine papillae. Towards the posterior end a single *vallate papilla* about the size of the head of a common pin occurs at each side, sunk in a sort of ditch to the level of the surrounding surface, and anterolateral to this appears a larger area covered by very fine oblique folds, whence is derived its name, *papilla foliata.* Sunk into the surfaces of the papillae are the microscopic taste buds.

93

5. Behind the base of the tongue a small, deep pit may be observed in each side of the pharynx, with a thickened mass of lymphoid tissue in its anterior wall. The latter masses are the *palatine tonsils,* the pits are the *tonsillar sinuses.*

6. The *epiglottis,* a prominent, curved, transverse fold stiffened by flexible fibrocartilage projects from the floor of the pharynx and guards the entrance to the respiratory tract.

7. The *nasopharynx* may now be opened by a longitudinal incision through the soft palate, which membrane ends just in front of the epiglottis. Anteriorly the nasopharynx is continuous with the two *nasal fossae* and in each lateral wall appears the small opening of the *auditory* or *Eustachian tube,* which connects the nasopharynx with the cavity of the middle ear.

8. The *larynx* may be examined in further detail if it is so desired. By cutting round the base of the tongue on the side still attached and severing the trachea in the lower part of the neck, these structures may be removed in a single piece. The *thyreoid gland* should be noted. It is a bilobed brown mass with a ventral connection of the two lobes applied to the trachea a little behind the larynx.

The larynx should then be separated from the remnants of the pharyngeal wall and cleaned by carefully scraping away the small muscles which conceal its flexible cartilages, especially dorsally.

(*a*) The *thyreoid cartilage* is the largest and surrounds the lateral and ventral aspects of the upper part of the larynx.

(*b*) The *cricoid cartilage* is a complete ring round the lower part of the larynx. Its dorsal portion expands into a broad plate, the *lamina,* which is attached by short firm ligaments to the posterodorsal angles of the thyreoid cartilage.

(*c*) The *arytenoid cartilages* are small, obliquely situated, curved structures applied to the anterolateral margins of the lamina of the cricoid.

(*d*) The *corniculate cartilages* are minute bodies, so small and soft as often to give difficulty in their recognition, lying one at the anterior tip of each arytenoid cartilage.

(*e*) The *epiglottic cartilage* is a thin, very flexible plate occupying the fold of mucous membrane that constitutes the epiglottis.

(*f*) The *vocal folds* may be observed by looking into the opening from the pharynx. They are vertical folds of the mucous membrane at each side of the laryngeal cavity and are poorly developed in the rabbit, often being flattened in the embalmed specimens so as to be unrecognizable if the larynx is opened.

CHAPTER XIX

CONTENTS OF THE ORBIT

A. Structures Associated with the Eye

THE eye is protected externally by the upper and lower lids and by the third eyelid, as pointed out in the chapter on external features. If these have not already been removed, the skin should be stripped off to the middorsal line, the lining (conjunctiva) of the lids being cut. The eyeball should be freed by carefully tearing the connective tissue attaching it to the rim of the orbit and the supraorbital process of the frontal bone should be broken away.

1. The opening of the *nasolacrimal duct* appears in the anterior part of the lining of the lower eyelid.

2. The *levator palpebrae superioris muscle* is an extremely thin sheet with its origin on the medial wall of the orbit and its insertion in the skin of the upper eyelid. It should be removed to expose the underlying structures.

3. The extrinsic muscles of the eye.

(*a*) The *superior oblique muscle* has its origin on the anterior margin of the optic foramen and passes dorsad close to the orbital wall to loop round a short ligamentous cord, the *trochlea*, from which the muscle extends obliquely caudolaterad to be inserted on the anterodorsal surface of the eye.

(*b*) The *inferior oblique muscle* is approximately parallel with the insertion portion of the superior oblique, passing from an origin on the lacrimal bone to an insertion on the posteroventral surface of the eye.

(*c*) The *superior rectus* has its origin on the upper margin of the optic foramen and runs anterolaterad to be inserted on the dorsal surface of the eye just behind the superior oblique.

(*d*) The *inferior rectus* also originates on the margin of the optic foramen and its insertion is on the ventral surface of the eye, overlapped by that of the inferior oblique.

(*e*) The *medial* and *lateral recti* originate from the margin of the foramen and are inserted on the anterior and posterior surfaces of the eye respectively.

(*f*) The *retractor oculi,* or *retractor bulbi,* is differentiated from the recti in mammals. It originates on the posterior margin of the foramen and partly surrounds the optic nerve, being inserted on the ventromedial part of the eye.

4. The *Harderian gland* is a large mass in the anterior part of the orbit. Its presence is associated with that of a well-developed third eyelid, on the internal surface of which its duct opens. It is peculiar in the rabbit and hare in consisting of two parts, the larger grey-red, the smaller usually whitish.

5. The *lacrimal gland* in the posterior end of the orbit is much smaller and usually darker.

6. An *infraorbital gland* related to the lacrimal lies in the ventral part of the orbit.

7. The *optic nerve* passes from the ventromedial surface of the eye directly to the optic foramen to enter the skull.

B. The Eye

The extrinsic muscles should be severed at their insertions and the optic nerve cut. The eyeball may then be divided into outer and inner hemispheres by a circular cut parallel with the edge of the coloured portion. The mass of transparent jelly within, the vitreous body, is best cut with scissors and the internal structure should be observed under water.

1. The *fibrous tunic* is the relatively thick, tough, outer layer of the whole eyeball. The greater part of it is opaque and white, the *sclera* or *sclerotic coat,* but over most of the normally exposed part of the eye it is transparent and colourless, the *cornea.*

2. The *vascular tunic* is the black layer just internal to the fibrous tunic. The greater part of this, lining the sclera, is the *chorioidea,* which is firmly fused with a thin inner sheet, the pigmented epithelium of the retina. The chorioidea is continuous with the *ciliary body,* a thicker, circular band containing smooth muscles and marked by radiating ridges, which surrounds the lens. The *iris* is also circular in the rabbit and projects from the inner margin of the ciliary body over the outer side of the lens, forming the coloured part visible through the cornea in the intact eye. The opening in the centre of the iris is the *pupil.*

3. The *retina* appears as a thin, milky-looking layer lining the wall of the eyeball. It is composed mainly of nerve-elements with their supporting structures and is the actually sensory part of the eye, continuous with the optic nerve. It is divisible into a very

thin *ciliary portion* applied to the internal surface of the ciliary body and a more extensive *optic* or *sensory portion* internal to the chorioidea.

A little posteroventral to the centre of the retina lies the *optic disc,* or "blind spot", where the fibres in the retina converge to turn mediad as the optic nerve.

4. The *lens* is a somewhat flattened, circular, hard, transparent body suspended by extremely fine colourless *zonular fibres* from the inner edge of the ciliary body. The lens focusses the light passing through it upon the retina, its curvature being slightly modifiable by varying pull of the ciliary muscles on the zonular fibres.

5. The *vitreous body* is a mass of colourless jelly filling the space surrounded by the retina and the lens.

6. The *aqueous humour occupies* the space between the lens and the cornea, which space is divided by the iris into an outer *anterior chamber* and an inner *posterior chamber* communicating through the pupil.

Chapter XX

THE SPINAL CORD AND SPINAL NERVES

The activities of all parts caudal to the head are controlled through the spinal cord, although in a few cases this influence may be modified by cranial nerves, such as the vagus or the spinal accessory. The spinal cord is an organ which receives nerve-impulses through afferent nerve-fibres and either transmits them directly to appropriate efferent nerve-fibres (simple reflex) or conveys them to

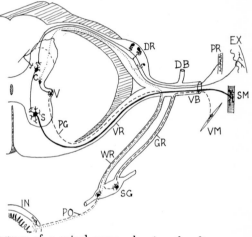

FIG. 25. Diagram of a spinal nerve, showing the direct central and peripheral connections of its fibres. C, connector neuron in grey matter of spinal cord; DB, dorsal branch of spinal nerve; DR, dorsal root with ganglion; EX, exteroceptive ending in skin; GR, grey ramus communicans; IN, intestine, with afferent and efferent nerve endings in its wall; PG, preganglionic visceral efferent neuron; PO, postganglionic visceral efferent neuron; PR, proprioceptive ending in a muscle spindle; S. somatic efferent neuron; SG, sympathetic ganglion; SM, ending of somatic efferent neuron in striated muscle; V, cell-body of visceral efferent neuron; VB, ventral branch of spinal nerve; VM, ending of visceral efferent fibre in smooth muscle; VR, ventral root;WR, white ramus communicans.

higher correlating centres in the brain, where they may influence more complex responses. It also conveys impulses from the brain to posterior efferent paths. Hence the spinal cord is composed of nerve-cell-bodies and nerve-fibres in very large numbers. The fibres may or may not be provided with white, fatty, myelin sheaths. As the fibres are grouped largely in the outer part of the cord, the tissue here has a white appearance due to these sheaths (white substance) and the cord as a whole is white. The cell-bodies with their shorter receptive processes and the points of connection (synapses) are mostly assembled internally in the *grey matter.*

It is desirable that the full extent of the spinal cord should be exposed. This may be accomplished by stripping off the muscles from the dorsal and dorsolateral aspects of the vertebral column and breaking away the vertebral arches with bone-forceps.

1. The *dura mater* is first exposed. It is a rather tough membrane completely surrounding the spinal cord but not attached to the bone of the vertebrae. The dura mater is the outermost of three membranes, the *meninges,* which invest the central nervous organs. Cutting it open reveals a much more delicate membrane intimately applied to the surface of the spinal cord and containing the finer blood-vessels for the latter. This membrane is the innermost meninx, the *pia mater.* Between it and the dura mater is a loose, somewhat spongy sheet, so fine that it is called the *arachnoidea* and is not readily recognized in a gross dissection.

Watery *cerebrospinal fluid* occupies the space between the meninges as well as the cavities in the central nervous organs during life.

2. The spinal cord is a massive, white tube of varying diameter. It is wide in the neck region (*cervical enlargement*), with the lower part of which the nerves of the fore limb are connected, narrower in the thoracic region, and wider again in the lumbar region (*lumbar enlargement*), where it is related to the nerves of the hind limb.

Near the middle of the sacrum, the spinal cord tapers rapidly and is replaced by a slender non-nervous thread, the *filum terminale,* which runs back through the more anterior caudal vertebrae. This arrangement is due to the spinal cord growing less rapidly than surrounding parts during the later stages of development.

The dorsal surface of the spinal cord is marked by a longitudinal groove, the *dorsal median sulcus,* which is most distinct anteriorly. The dorsal roots of the spinal nerves enter the cord a short distance lateral to this sulcus.

3. The *first spinal nerve* at each side enters the vertebral canal behind the skull and each succeeding one enters behind the corresponding vertebra. Thus there are eight *cervical nerves,* including the first and the seven which lie behind the seven cervical vertebrae.

Twelve *thoracic,* seven *lumbar,* four *sacral,* and six *caudal* nerves then occur in regular sequence.

The relatively slower growth of the spinal cord which produced the filum terminale also resulted in the moving of the connections of the more posterior nerves to levels cephalic to their emergence from the vertebral column so that they run obliquely within the canal, a group of them coursing at each side of the filum terminale.

4. The *roots* of a single nerve should be examined. For this purpose the lateral parts of two adjacent vertebral arches should be carefully broken away so as to expose the nerve between them, preferably in the thoracic region. The dura mater must be removed from the roots and these may be further cleared by stripping away the pia mater but are liable to be broken off if this is not done very carefully.

The nerve is connected with the spinal cord by a *dorsal root* and a *ventral root,* the latter directly beneath the former, each composed of a series of rootlets converging in fan-like form to the compact nerve. The dorsal root is made up of afferent fibres, the ventral one of efferent fibres. Where the rootlets of the dorsal root unite laterally there is a swelling, the *dorsal root ganglion* or *spinal ganglion,* and the ventral root joins the dorsal one just beyond this, close to the intervertebral foramen.

The nerve thus constituted almost at once breaks into three primary branches, a *dorsal ramus* to the muscles and skin of the back, a larger *ventral ramus* to the rest of the muscles and skin, and a very slender *ramus communicans* to the sympathetic trunk for innervation of the viscera. Each branch contains both afferent and efferent fibres.

5. If a small piece of the spinal cord is removed by cutting transversely, the cut surface may be examined with a magnifying glass or, better, stained sections may be studied at a low magnification.

The cord is seen to be a tube with a minute central canal and an extremely thick wall. Round the canal is *grey matter* which in transverse section has roughly the form of the letter H, and outside this is a thick layer of *white matter.* The white matter is divided into right and left halves by the dorsal median sulcus, already noted on the surface, and a corresponding *ventral median fissure.*

CHAPTER XXI

THE BRAIN

EXAMINATION of the brain requires first the opening of the skull, which should be performed with bone-forceps after the soft tissues have been cleared away. It may be commenced either from behind or from in front, a convenient approach being to cut across the roof of the cranium between the front parts of the orbits, then to break away the supraoccipital processes and cut through the cranial wall along each side so that pieces of the roof can be pried off. This procedure is continued back to the level of the ears. The temporal portion of the skull should be crushed with the points of the forceps and picked away in small pieces so as not to destroy the paraflocculus, a stalked portion of the brain which projects laterad with the bone fitting closely round it. The remainder of the roof and the lateral walls of the brain-case being now removed, the brain may be raised gently and the nerve-roots and fibrous attachments may be cut *with scissors* as close to the skull as possible. Finally the spinal cord should be severed at about the second or third cervical segment and the brain should be lifted out. If it is to be kept for study in a later period, it should be preserved in 50% alcohol.

The pituitary gland will have remained sunk in the floor of the brain-case, whence it may be removed for examination.

1. The *meninges,* which were observed surrounding the spinal cord, are continued over the brain. The dura mater, however, is firmly adherent to the inner surface of the cranium, instead of lying loosely internal to the bone as it does in the vertebral column. Folds extend into the grooves between certain main divisions of the brain and it is often convenient to cut these with scissors in order to remove the dura mater.

2. The primary divisions of the brain are three, which appear early in embryonic history and are known as the *forebrain* (prosencephalon), *midbrain* (mesencephalon), and *hindbrain* (rhombencephalon). Each has become considerably elaborated in form, the forebrain most and the midbrain least, but they are still recognized in the adult. The forebrain is considered to be subdivisible

101

into the endbrain (telencephalon) and the 'tweenbrain (diencephalon). The hindbrain also is divided into two, the pons plus cerebellum (metencephalon) and the medulla oblongata (myelencephalon).

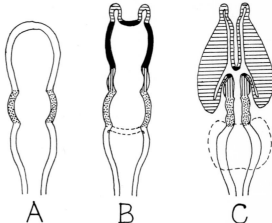

A   B   C

Fig. 26. Diagrams of horizontal sections through the brain, A in an early embryo, B in a prototypical vertebrate, C in a rabbit. The mesencephalon is stippled. In B and C the cerebellum (metencephalon) is indicated by broken outlines, the 'tweenbrain (diencephalon) by vertical hatching, the unevaginated part of the endbrain (telencephalon medium) in solid black, and the evaginated part of the endbrain (olfactory bulbs and cerebral hemispheres) by horizontal hatching.

3. The *hindbrain* is the direct continuation forward of the spinal cord, there being no obvious boundary between them.

(*a*) The *cerebellum* is the conspicuous dorsal portion of the hindbrain. It is composed of numerous transverse folds covered with grey matter, the *cerebellar cortex*. Various subdivisions are recognizable and at each side projects the prominent, stalked *paraflocculus*. The cerebellum is concerned in muscular coordination, the maintenance of muscle-tone, and equilibration.

(*b*) The *cerebellar peduncles* form a rather massive connection at each side between the cerebellum and the parts of the brain ventral to it. They are composed of nerve-fibres entering and leaving the cerebellum. Severing the peduncles and the thin membranes under the cerebellum (medullary vela — (*c*) and (*d*)below) makes it possible to remove the cerebellum entirely.

(*c*) The *pons* and the cerebellum together constitute the metencephalon. The pons is the more anterior portion of the hindbrain, directly continuous with the medulla oblongata behind and lying ventral to most of the cerebellum. It is distinguished mainly by a large superficial mass of transverse nerve-fibres forming a prominent elevation on its lateral and ventral surfaces. This *pontine tract* is continuous at each side with the middle peduncle of the cerebellum and is composed of fibres conveying into the cerebellar cortex impulses that have been transmitted to them from the cerebral cortex.

The hindbrain contains a wide, lozenge-shaped cavity, the *fourth ventricle*, continuous with the central canal of the spinal cord. The anterior part of this ventricle lies in the region of the pons, where it tapers towards the narrower cavity in the midbrain. Its thin roof is the *anterior medullary velum*. The posterior edge of the anterior medullary velum and the anterior edge of the posterior medullary velum are both attached to the under surface of the cerebellum, so that they will have been cut or torn in its removal.

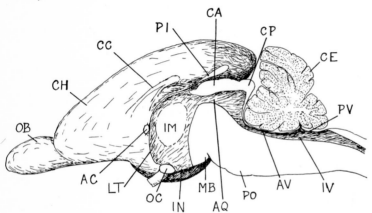

FIG. 27. Median section of the brain. AC, anterior commissure; AQ, cerebral aqueduct; AV, anterior medullary velum; CA, anterior colliculus; CC, corpus callosum; CE, cerebellum; CH, cerebral hemisphere; CP, posterior colliculus; IM, intermediate mass; IN, infundibulum; IV, fourth ventricle; LT, terminal lamina; MB, mamillary body; OB, olfactory bulb; OC, optic chiasma; PI, pineal body; PO, pons; PV, posterior medullary velum.

(*d*) The *medulla oblongata* (myelencephalon) appears like a forward expansion of the spinal cord. Its massive lateral and ventral walls contain the connections of the more posterior cranial nerves (which are described below) and large bundles of nerve-fibres running between more anterior and more posterior parts of the central nervous system. Thus they include reflex centres, especially for the head region; centres for auditory, equilibratory, gustatory, and other sensory impulses; centres for correlation of impulses received; the respiratory centre; and extensive conduction pathways.

The roof of the expanded ventricle is a very thin membrane, the *posterior medullary velum,* containing a network of fine blood-vessels, the *posterior chorioid plexus,* and largely overlapped by the cerebellum.

(e) Most of the cranial nerves connect with the hindbrain.

(i) The *hypoglossal,* or twelfth cranial nerve, a motor nerve for the tongue, emerges from the ventral surface of the posterior part of the medulla oblongata by a row of rootlets emerging in line with the ventral roots of the spinal nerves. Thus each row is somewhat lateral to the ventral median fissure, which continues from the spinal cord to the caudal edge of the pons.

(ii) The *accessory* (eleventh), the *vagus* (tenth), and the *glossopharyngeal* (ninth) nerves emerge as a continuous series of rootlets along the lateral surface of the medulla oblongata. The glossopharyngeal and the vagus are mixed nerves, that is, they contain both afferent and efferent fibres. The efferent fibres belong to the parasympathetic group. They are distributed to parts of the digestive, respiratory, and circulatory systems, fibres of the vagus going to the alimentary canal as far as the ascending colon, as well as to its glands, to the lungs and bronchi, and to the heart. The accessory nerve has a trunk which extends back between the dorsal and ventral roots of the spinal nerves as far as the fifth cervical. It has apparently been formed by the assembling of certain efferent fibres from the vagus and from the more anterior spinal nerves and it supplies muscles of the throat and of the shoulder.

(iii) The *acoustic,* or eighth cranial nerve connects with the dorsolateral angle of the oblongata just behind the cerebellar peduncles, carrying auditory and equilibratory impulses from the internal ear. A slight swelling extending dorsomediad behind the peduncle is the acoustic tubercle, in which many of the auditory fibres end.

(iv) The *facial,* or seventh cranial nerve joins the brain close to and just in front of the acoustic nerve. It contains the motor fibres controlling the facial muscles and a smaller group of afferent (largely gustatory) components.

(v) The *abducent,* or sixth cranial nerve is very slender, being composed of the motor fibres for only one of the extrinsic muscles of the eye (the lateral rectus, which abducts the eye). It rises on the ventral surface of the oblongata anteriorly, in line with the more posterior hypoglossal nerve.

(vi) The *trigeminal*, or fifth cranial nerve includes a large sensory root from the skin of the face and a smaller motor root for the muscles of mastication. These roots penetrate the lateral part of the pons and the large nerve extends almost directly forward at first. Its name is derived from the fact that it divides into three main branches.

(vii) The *trochlear*, or fourth cranial nerve emerges at the boundary between hindbrain and midbrain. It is peculiar in that it emerges from the dorsal surface, just where the anterior medullary velum is connected to the midbrain, and curves down over the lateral surface. The trochlear is a motor nerve for the superior oblique muscle of the eye and gets its name from the fact that this muscle passes over a trochlea (p. 95).

4. The *midbrain* lies directly anterior to the hindbrain.

(a) The dorsal side rises above the level of the medulla oblongata and pons and appears as two pairs of rounded masses, the *corpora quadrigemina*. The posterior pair of these, the *inferior colliculi*, is the smaller and is occupied by centres where auditory impulses are correlated with a great variety of other sensory impulses. The considerably larger *superior colliculi* in front contain visual correlation centres and correspond with the optic lobes of lower vertebrates.

(b) The *cerebral peduncles* are a pair of broad, longitudinal bands of nerve-fibres which form the more restricted ventral surface of the midbrain. Their component fibres are derived from the cerebral cortex and convey impulses to the pons, the medulla oblongata, and the spinal cord.

(c) The *oculomotor*, or third cranial nerve emerges through each cerebral peduncle. It is a motor nerve to the extrinsic muscles of the eye not innervated by the abducent or the trochlear nerve.

5. The *forebrain* is the largest of the three primary divisions of the brain. It comprises an unpaired part, the *'tweenbrain* (diencephalon), continuous caudally with the midbrain, and, in front of the 'tweenbrain, the *endbrain* (telencephalon), composed of the paired cerebral hemispheres, with a very small interconnecting portion.

(a) The 'tweenbrain is concealed from above by the overlapping cerebral hemispheres, the caudal ends of which should be gently raised and spread apart. This procedure will reveal a massive region with a partly membranous roof to which a small, stalked body is attached.

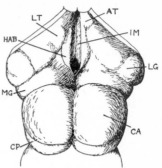

Fig. 28. Dorsal view of the 'tweenbrain and the midbrain. AT, anterior tubercle of the thalamus; CA, anterior colliculus of the midbrain; CP, posterior colliculus of the midbrain; HAB, habenula; IM, intermediate mass, bridging third ventricle; LG, lateral geniculate body; LT, lateral tubercle of the thalamus; MG; medial geniculate body.

(i) The *pineal body* or *gland* is the stalked body just mentioned, which projects backwards to lie in the groove between the superior colliculi. It is an endocrine gland concerning the functions of which little is yet known. The pineal body should be torn away, carrying with it the membranous roof of the 'tweenbrain, which contains another chorioid plexus (chorioid plexus of the third ventricle).

(ii) The 'tweenbrain, though described above as unpaired, is now seen to be composed of paired masses lying at each side of a narrow, median cleft, the *third ventricle*, from which the membranous roof has just been removed. This is connected with the fourth ventricle behind by a narrow passage through the midbrain and with paired ventricles (counted as the first two) in the cerebral hemispheres.

(iii) The thick mass of nervous tissue at each side of the ventricle shows several more or less distinct eminences. The most lateral part is the *lateral geniculate body*, which receives the endings of many of the fibres from the eyes and transmits their impulses to the cerebral cortex.

A less prominent *medial geniculate body* just caudomedial to this is a corresponding centre for auditory impulses to be relayed to the cortex.

(iv) The cut ends of the *optic*, or second cranial nerves should appear on the ventral surface. These nerves interlace in the median plane, many fibres passing from one side to the other and thus forming a prominent cross, the *optic chiasma.* From the chiasma the optic fibres continue without interruption as the *optic tract* extending caudodorsad over the surface to the lateral geniculate body and the superior colliculus, in one or other of which they terminate.

(v) The *pituitary body* (hypophysis) is attached to the ventral surface of the brain just behind the optic chiasma but is broken off unless special precautions have been taken in removing it from the skull. It is a small, rounded, endocrine gland of great importance in regulating many activities of the organs in the body, both directly and by acting on other endocrine glands. It is of outstanding importance for normal growth and development. The former position of the lost pituitary body is indicated by a small, median slit, which is the cavity of its hollow, broken stalk (infundibulum, Fig. 27).

(vi) The *tuber cinereum* is the grey tissue surrounding the slit just mentioned. It is part of the *hypothalamus,* a ventral portion of the 'tweenbrain containing complex centres for regulation of vegetative functions of the body, such as the maintenance of uniform temperature, water-metabolism, etc..

(vii) The *mamillary body* projects conspicuously behind the tuber cinereum and is also part of the hypothalamus. It is a region for correlation in which olfactory and visceral connections play a predominant part.

(*b*) The endbrain comprises all of the brain in front of the parts just described.

(i) The *cerebral hemispheres* are two large, roughly pear-shaped expansions, each hollow, thick-walled, and having an outer layer of grey matter, the *cerebral cortex.* This cortex is of oustanding importance as containing the highest centres for influencing the activities of other parts of the nervous system and, through them, of the animal as a whole. In mammals with large brains the cerebral cortex becomes folded but in the rabbit it remains nearly smooth.

(ii) The *longitudinal cerebral fissure* separates the two hemispheres in the median plane.

(iii) The *olfactory bulb* is a somewhat ovoid mass at the cephalic end of each cerebral hemisphere. It receives the endings of the many separate threads constituting the *olfactory,* or first cranial nerve.

(iv) If observed laterally or ventrally, the olfactory bulb is seen to be continued caudad by a narrower band which expands into the ventral part of the cerebral hemisphere, the *pyriform lobe*. This, the olfactory portion of the hemisphere, is delimited from the non-olfactory portion above it by a longitudinal groove, the *limbic* or *rhinal fissure*.

(v) The two cerebral hemispheres are interconnected by several transverse bands of nerve-fibres, or *commissures*. The largest of these, one peculiar to mammals, is the *corpus callosum*, which connects the cortex of each hemisphere with that of the other. It may be observed by pulling apart the hemispheres so as to open up the longitudinal cerebral fissure.

(vi) By removal of a piece of the dorsal wall of one hemisphere the thickness of the cortex, the layer of white matter beneath it, and the cavity within (*lateral ventricle*) may be seen.

6. The main blood vessels of the brain run through the subarachnoid space, their smaller branches in the pia mater, from which they penetrate the nervous tissue. The larger veins are mostly dorsal and empty into sinuses in the dura mater. The larger arteries are ventral.

(*a*) The *basilar artery*, an unpaired median vessel on the ventral surface of the medulla oblongata, receives blood caudally from the paired vertebral arteries, branches of the subclavian. Irregular superficial and deep branches include a pair of *inferior cerebellar arteries*, and at the rostral edge of the pons the trunk bifurcates to form the posterior cerebral arteries.

(*b*) The paired *posterior cerebral artery* supplies the diencephalon and the caudal portion of the cerebral hemisphere. It also gives off a large *superior cerebellar artery* and a short, rostrally-directed, *posterior communicating artery*. The latter connects with the internal carotid.

(*c*) The *internal carotid artery* is a continuation of the common carotid (p. 80) and, having penetrated the base of the skull, appears as a cut stump at each side of the tuber cinereum.

(*d*) The internal carotid turns rostrad and divides into the *middle cerebral artery*, to the lateral and dorsal parts of the cerebral hemisphere, and the *anterior cerebral artery*, to the rostroventral part of the hemisphere and the olfactory bulb. The pair of anterior cerebral arteries unites as a short common trunk (where an anterior communicating artery occurs in man) which redivides to the medial surfaces of the hemispheres. A complete anastomotic loop, the *circle of Willis*, is thus formed by the anterior cerebral, internal carotid, posterior communicating, and posterior cerebral arteries.

APPENDIX

HEAD AND NECK

REMOVE the skin from the head, observing the *platysma muscle,* a thin sheet under the skin, inserted on that of the cheek and usually remaining attached to it. The platysma is part of the same layer as the cutaneous maximus of the abdomen. Its nerve supply, like that of the facial muscles, is through the seventh cranial nerve.

1. *Superficial structures*

(a) The *masseter muscle* (origin: the zygomatic arch) lies on the lateral surface of the mandible, inserted on the angle. A second muscle of mastication, the *pterygoideus (external* and *internal)* lies on the medial surface of the mandible.

(b) *Salivary glands*

(i) *Parotid gland* lies directly behind the angle of the mandible. The *parotid duct* crosses the masseter along with branches of the facial nerve and opens into the oral cavity.

(ii) *Submaxillary* (better *Submandibular*) *gland,* more compact, lies at the medial side of the ventral margin of the angle of the mandible. Its duct runs dorsad and slightly forward to enter the floor of the mouth.

(iii) (A third salivary gland, the *sublingual,* not to be dissected at present, lies beneath the tongue.)

(c) The *digastricus muscle* is just medial to the angle of the mandible, overlapping the internal pterygoid. Origin: by a long concealed tendon from the base of the skull. Insertion: on the anterior portion of the medial surface of the mandible. It is the depressor of the lower jaw.

(d) The *mylohyoideus muscles,* one on either side, form a transverse sheet between the mandibles, from which they originate. They are inserted on the hyoid bone and raise the floor of the mouth.

(e) The *stylohyoideus major muscle.* Origin: Jugular process of the occipital bone, beside the digastricus. Insertion: tip of the greater horn of the hyoid.

(f) The *sternomastoideus muscle* has its origin on the manubrium sterni and is inserted on the mastoid process of the skull. Singly, it turns the head and depresses the snout. The pair, acting together, depresses the snout.

109

(g) The *sternohyoideus muscle*. Those of the two sides lie close together on the midventral line of the neck and have a common origin on the anterior portion of the sternum. Insertion is on the greater cornu of the hyoid. The two should be separated along the midline and divided.

(h) The *sternothyreoideus muscle*. Origin in common with the above. Insertion on the lateral plate of the thyreoid cartilage of the larynx. The *thyreohoideus muscle* is a continuation of the sternothyreoid from thyreoid cartilage to hyoid.

2. *Deeper structures*

(a) The *trachea* is the tube which carries air from the larynx to the lungs. Cartilaginous *tracheal rings* in its wall, incomplete dorsally, prevent its collapse.

(b) The heavy, annular, *cricoid cartilage* is just anterior to the first tracheal ring. In front of it is the broader, saddle-shaped, *thyreoid cartilage* of the larynx.

(c) Dorso-lateral to the thyreoid cartilage, an elongate body, the *deep cervical lymph gland*, lies close to the *internal jugular vein*.

(d) The *thyreoid gland* is composed of lateral masses on either side of the trachea, behind the cricoid cartilage, the two being connected ventrally by a very thin isthmus.

(e) The *common carotid artery* runs along the side of the trachea to the head. Branches are the *superior thyreoid artery* to the thyreoid gland and the *laryngeal artery* to the larynx and related muscles.

(f) The *internal jugular vein*, lateral to the common carotid artery, passing close to the deep cervical lymph gland, returns blood from the head to the heart.

(g) The *vagus nerve* lies lateral to the common carotid artery, between the latter and the internal jugular vein. It is the largest of four nerves (ramus descendens hypoglossi, cervical portion of the sympathetic trunk, vagus, and ramus cardiacus vagi or depressor nerve) accompanying the carotid, and is both sensory and motor. It is distributed to the larynx, the trachea, the lungs, the digestive tract, and the heart. Close to the skull it has an enlargement, the *ganglion nodosum*. The ramus cardiacus (p. 86, sec. 3) runs dorsal to the common carotid artery.

(h) The sympathetic trunk, with its superior and inferior cervical ganglia, is described on page 86 (sec. 4).

(i) The oesophagus, dorsal to the trachea, is the muscular tube that conveys material from the pharynx to the stomach.

INDEX

DATE DUE

ICL 3-4-82			
GAYLORD			PRINTED IN U.S.A.